Discussions in Patient Management

STROKE

Discussions in Patient Management

STROKE

By

LOWELL G. LUBIC, M.D.
Chief of Neurology
Montefiore Hospital;
Clinical Associate Professor of Neurology
University of Pittsburgh
Pittsburgh, Pennsylvania

and

HARRY P. PALKOVITZ, M.D.
Chief of Neurology
Shadyside Hospital;
Clinical Assistant Professor of Neurology
University of Pittsburgh
Pittsburgh, Pennsylvania

Medical Examination Publishing Co., Inc.
an Excerpta Medica company

969 Stewart Avenue • Garden City, New York 11530

Library of Congress Card Number
79-88044

ISBN 0-87488-893-X

May, 1979

Printed in the United States of America

SIMULTANEOUSLY PUBLISHED IN:

Europe	:	HANS HUBER PUBLISHERS Bern, Switzerland
Japan	:	IGAKU SHOIN Ltd. Tokyo, Japan
Mexico, Central America, and South America (except Brazil)	:	EDITORIAL EL MANUAL MODERNO Mexico City, Mexico
South and East Asia	:	TOPPAN COMPANY (S) Pte. Ltd. Singapore
United Kingdom	:	HENRY KIMPTON PUBLISHERS London, England

PREFACE

The explosive technological advances in platelet antagonists, computerized tomography scanning of the brain, arteriography, and vascular surgery have allowed us to develop a firm approach to the management of occlusive cerebrovascular disease. We believe this book represents a holistic modern approach to these unique problems.

While there are many books published on the topic of ischemic cerebrovascular disease, the purpose of this book is to present a concise and thorough discussion of the management of patients with occlusive cerebrovascular disease. It presents the recommended course of therapy when there is general agreement and presents alternatives when there is considerable disagreement. In the latter situation, the authors attempt to provide their readers a critical review of pertinent literature and discussions with experienced colleagues, based on data obtained from thirty years of active practice in clinical neurology.

The Authors

ACKNOWLEDGMENTS

We wish to thank Ms. Cynthia Haubelt, Ms. Nancy Reedy, Ms. Martha Wisenauer, and Ms. Donna Fazio for typing the manuscript. We also wish to thank Mr. Thomas Kruper for the illustrations.

Contents

notice

The editor(s) and/or author(s) and the publisher of this book have made every effort to ensure that all therapeutic modalities that are recommended are in accordance with accepted standards at the time of publication.

The drugs specified within this book may not have specific approval by the Food and Drug Administration in regard to the indications and dosages that are recommended by the editor(s) and/or author(s). The manufacturer's package insert is the best source of current prescribing information.

CHAPTER I:

TRANSIENT ISCHEMIC ATTACKS

PART ONE: CAROTID SYSTEMS

GENERAL INFORMATION

In the past twenty years, transient ischemic attacks have aroused a great deal of interest in the medical profession because they produce a warning of impending stroke in certain patients. About 1.2 million completed strokes occur annually in the United States; about three-fourths, or 900, 000 are preceded by transient ischemic attacks. About one-third of patients with defined transient ischemic attacks will have a completed stroke within one year.[1, 2]

The patients most likely to go on to a completed stroke are those with numerous transient ischemic attacks of the carotid system and those with symptoms and signs involving both vertebral-basilar and carotid system.[3]

Platelet-fibrin emboli are the most common cause of transient ischemic attacks in the carotid system. Less common are atheromatous (cholesterol) emboli. The atherosclerotic lesions that produce the emboli are most commonly located at the bifurcation of the common carotid artery into the internal and external carotid artery. Less common areas would be at the carotid syphon intracranially, and at the origin of the left common carotid artery and innominate artery from the aortic arch. The bifurcation of the innominate artery into the common carotid artery and the subclavian artery on the right are less common sites. These atherosclerotic plaques can narrow the <u>lumen</u> of the common carotid, the internal carotid, or external carotid arteries, or on occasion, can consist of ulcerated plaques that do not narrow the lumen of the vessels (Figure 1.1).

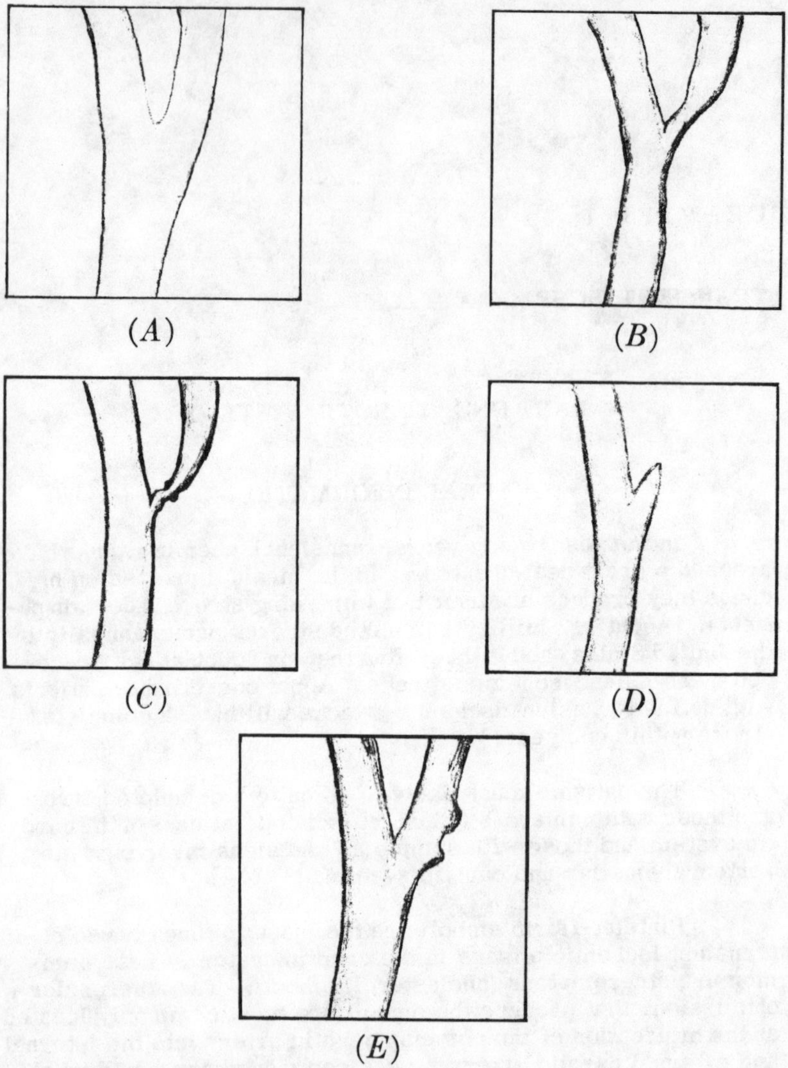

FIG. 1.1 (A) Normal bifuraction of common carotid artery into the internal carotid artery and external carotid artery; (B) Moderate narrowing of the internal carotid artery by a stenosing plaque (greater than 50%); (C) Severe narrowing of the internal carotid artery by a stenosing plaque (greater than 95%); (D) Total occlusion of the internal carotid artery; (E) Ulcerating plaques of the internal carotid artery without stenosis

Some specialists involved in carotid vascular disease are impressed by the degree of stenosis present, saying that the narrowing in the internal carotid artery system must be greater than 50% to be significant.[4] It is probably true that the narrowing of the internal carotid lumen must be greater than 95% to cause any significant decrease in the ipsilateral carotid blood flow; more likely the narrowing atherosclerotic plaques have ulcers or irregularities on the surface that attract platelet-fibrin clots which are subsequently showered into the ipsilateral carotid circulation; this implies that the degree of stenosis of the carotid lumen is not of primary importance other than it will lead with time to total occlusion of the common or internal carotid artery. No one disagrees that the ulcerated plaque is a potential nidus for platelet-fibrin emboli that can subsequently shower the involved internal carotid artery circulation.[5]

DIFFERENTIAL DIAGNOSIS

The single most important step for the physician is to accurately diagnose transient ischemic attacks. Incorrect diagnoses lead to unnecessary tests and improper therapy.

A transient ischemic attack always has a sudden onset and usually reaches its maximum intensity in two to five minutes. By definition, all of the symptoms and signs must be gone within twenty-four hours; most of the symptoms usually disappear rapidly within two to thirty minutes.[6] If the symptoms and signs persist beyond twenty-four hours, the diagnosis becomes changed to a completed stroke. It is apparent that twenty-four hours represents an arbitrary time limit that has no real significance other than to indicate a brief ischemic episode which was relatively benign in that it did not produce a fixed neurological deficit.

Diagnosis will depend strongly on getting an accurate history from the patient. In general, it is rare to see a patient during a transient ischemic attack. However, a skilled physician can increase the likelihood of a correct diagnosis if he is fortunate enough to be present during an attack. As you might expect, large studies have shown that during an attack the patient has more symptoms and signs than he would generally describe if the physician were not present.[7] In general, the attacks seen by a physician are of longer duration than the classic transient ischemic episodes. With carotid system transient ischemic attacks, these symptoms and signs could consist of an aphasic reaction, i.e., trouble with writing, reading, calculating, speaking, and understanding the spoken word; a central facial paresis, unilateral Babinski sign, retinal emboli, either fibrin platelet or cholesterol in type, homonymous hemianopia, hemiparesis, monoparesis, and sensory changes in one arm or leg or both.[8,9,10]

Be very cautious in interpreting histories from elderly patients with dementia and from patients who are known to be poor historians. Try not to be suggestive when obtaining a history. The accuracy of the diagnosis will increase if the patient's symptoms are stereotyped with each transient ischemic episode. In many cases, the ultimate diagnosis can only be made after several recurrent attacks. The patient's ability to perceive his symptoms will improve with repetitive episodes.

The most common symptom of a carotid transient ischemic attack is monocular blindness or monocular blurring of vision (amaurosis fugax). Sometimes the blurring of vision comes down like a curtain from superiorly to inferiorly, and sometimes it is a diffuse sudden blurring and sometimes it is a partial blurring of vision in a previously normal eye. If the visual loss is associated with weakness or numbness of the opposite extremities, the diagnosis of carotid disease is almost a certainty.

Do not confuse bright or colored scintillating scotoma with amaurosis fugax; the former are often associated with migrainous states. In addition, the migraine attacks are often followed by a severe headache, which is very rare with amaurosis fugax.

The physician must recognize that homonymous hemianopia is often interpreted by the patient as a loss of vision in one eye. Always ask the patient what happened if he closed the involved eye; was there any blurring or abnormal vision in the other eye? The presence of some visual defect in the opposite eye suggests that the visual problem represents a homonymous hemianopia. The latter symptoms can occur both with carotid or vertebral basilar ischemia and by itself will not distinguish which system is involved. The presence of dysphasia (aphasic disorder) is an unequivocal sign of carotid artery disease. In a right-handed patient the diagnosis of left carotid disease will be correct in over 95% of the cases. If the patient is left-handed, dysphasia by itself will not determine which carotid system is involved. Do not confuse dysphasia (aphasic reaction) with dysarthria; the latter represents a distortion of speech quality and can occur in both carotid or vertebral basilar ischemic attacks.

With receptive aphasia, the patient will have trouble understanding what is said to him. If there is a witness present, he will state that the patient was alert but did not seem to comprehend speech or could not carry out simple directions. In general, with receptive aphasia, the patient is unable to read; he may also state that he can think of a word but is unable to speak that word. This suggests that he was having an anomic aphasic reaction which is commonly seen with posterior aphasias originating in the temporal lobe. The patient may also have difficulty with calculations during an aphasic reaction.

With dysarthria, the patient will understand everything that is said to him but his speech will not be clear. He may have trouble pronouncing certain words but the syntax is correct. The deficit with dysarthria is due to weakness or incoordination in the muscles of articulation. The patient with an anomic aphasia will have difficulty coming up with key words in his sentence structure. There will be a hesitancy when he speaks, particularly when he is groping for a key word to complete his sentence.

If a patient cannot speak at all, this suggests a motor apraxia or a Broca's aphasia. The patient will be able to understand everything that is said to him and he will be able to carry out directions, but he will not be able to speak. In addition, with most motor aphasias, the patient is unable to write. Motor aphasias are much less common than receptive aphasias. In many patients, there will be a global aphasia indicating that the patient is unable to understand what is said to him and is unable to articulate words.

Careful questioning is indicated to rule out confusional states which do <u>not</u> represent carotid transient ischemic attacks. With psychomotor seizures, the patients often have an aura that precedes the attack. The aura can consist of rising epigastric sensation; formed or unformed visual hallucinations; unpleasant odors; unpleasant tastes; and noises which are interpreted as sounds in both ears. In addition, during the attack, the patient does not understand what is said to him; and he will have partial or complete amnesia for the episode. The patient with transient ischemic attacks in the carotid system does not have amnesic problems. After the psychomotor seizure, the patient is often tired and sometimes has urinary incontinence and postictal confusion for a short period of time. These symptoms are not seen with carotid transient ischemic attacks. During the convulsion itself, the patient may have automatic movements of the face, tongue, lips, or of the extremities which clearly indicate that he is having a psychomotor seizure.

The other common symptoms seen with carotid transient ischemic attacks are subjective numbness or paresthesias and/or weakness involving the contralateral face, arm, and leg. The numbness and weakness can occur together or separately. There is usually no spread or "march" effect with the numbness or weakness. All of the symptoms develop at one time. The weakness is often referred to as a heaviness or clumsiness of the extremity. The clumsiness must be differentiated from cerebellar ataxia, which would rarely occur in one arm and exclude the ipsilateral leg. In general, the patients with appendicular cerebellar ataxia do not complain of weakness or heaviness but describe clumsiness of their extremities. If the weakness occurs primarily in the leg, the patient will complain of difficulty with walking. Again, this must be differentiated from truncal ataxia that is seen with vertebral basilar disease. The latter is described by the patient as a feeling as if he is walking like a drunk. The patient with weakness in the leg will complain that the problem lies primarily in one leg and will not describe the feeling as if he is drunk. The numbness can be described by the patient as a pins and needles sensation or a numbing sensation. In addition, sometimes he will state that when he touches or rubs the involved extremity it will feel different from the opposite extremity.

Despite a careful history, the physician may have difficulty in separating appendicular ataxia from weakness in the extremities. Here, the association of other neurological symptoms may aid in the differential diagnosis.

Since most of the attacks are of brief duration, the physician may not be able to make the diagnosis from the original attack. He will have to re-evaluate the patient at a later date when the attacks recur. In these cases, the physician should instruct the patient how to differentiate weakness from ataxia. Tell him to hold his hands out in the prime outstretched position and see if one arm will drift down; tell him to sit in a chair and hold up both legs to see if one drifts down. Tell him to squeeze any object with both hands to see if there is a difference in the strength of his hand grip. These are all signs which point to pyramidal weakness in the involved extremities. Finally, show him how to test for ataxia. Have him perform the finger-to-nose test on both sides and then compare the sides. If the leg is involved, have him place one heel onto the opposite knee and run it down the shin to the ankle and then back up again. If the patient carries out these tests, the physician should be able, from the history obtained, to differentiate cerebellar ataxia from weakness. If the patient has trouble with speaking or understanding, ask him to try to read or write or calculate during the episode, as this may solidify the diagnosis of an aphasic disorder. With a reasonably intelligent patient, these tests should be useful in differentiating posterior circulation disease from anterior circulation disease, particularly if the attack lasts for several minutes.

Try not to confuse the patients with classic migraine headaches, who have a prolonged aura with those patients who have transient ischemic attacks. The migraine patient complains of weakness or numbness in the arm or leg. This weakness and numbness often has a spread or "march" quality which rarely occurs in transient ischemic attacks. The aura of a migraine may last from several minutes to hours and are most often followed by a severe headache usually on the contralateral side. There is often a family history of migraine. The patients are usually in an age group that is younger than those seen with transient ischemic attacks. With the migraine headache, the patients often have associated photophobia and vomiting.

Focal jacksonian seizures almost always have a "march" quality to them. The symptom will spread from the hand to the face to the arm and then to the leg. Sometimes this represents a clonic convulsive seizure and sometimes it represents a sensory jacksonian seizure which is characterized by paresthesias spreading in a "march" quality described above. With clonic movements, the differentiation becomes easy, but with jacksonian sensory seizures, the differentiation will sometimes be difficult unless one is able to establish a definite march pattern as previously described.

If the physician is present during the attack, he can quickly diagnose an aphasic disorder. First he must establish that the patient is alert and not confused. He should then give him several simple commands to carry out, such as touch your nose, close your eyes, take your left hand and touch your right knee. If he is able to carry out these directions, he does not have a significant receptive aphasia. Then ask him to repeat several phrases; if he repeats them adequately, he does not have a significant motor aphasia. Show him several objects such as a pencil, eraser, key, tie, and ask him to name them. This will rule out any significant anomic aphasia. If time permits, ask the patient to read or write. This quick survey will give the physician the ability to diagnose motor or receptive aphasia in patients with transient ischemic attacks of the carotid system. The weakness in the extremities can be easily perceived by the usual testing for strength and dexterity. Numbness of paresthesias in the patient is subjective and often not associated with objective neurological changes to pin, touch, stereognosis, or position sense. It is important for you to ask the patient if the sensory stimuli applied to the involved extremity or extremities feels different than the opposite side.

With amaurosis fugax, the physician should observe the fundi for platelet-fibrin emboli or for cholesterol emboli. The platelet-fibrin emboli are lodged in the retinal arterioles and have a gray-white color to them. The cholesterol emboli are highly refractory and project a bright color with the ophthalmoscope. The cholesterol emboli will usually stay in the retinal artery circulation longer than the platelet-fibrin emboli, and do not impair the blood flow through the involved vessel.

Gross visual field testing can be done at the time of the episode to distinguish whether the visual loss is primarily in one eye or represents some type of homonymous defect. The longer the attack lasts, the easier it will be for the physician to accurately diagnose carotid ischemic signs. During the attack, the pulse should be recorded for rate and rhythm and the heart auscultated. It is important to determine if any cardiac problem is present, particularly an arrhythmia, which could precipitate the transient ischemic episode. Blood pressure should be taken in both arms.

Cardiac arrhythmias can cause a decrease in cardiac output because of either profound tachycardia or profound bradycardia. In a patient with a moderate degree of carotid stenosis, the decreased cardiac output may lead to a hemodynamic ischemia of the involved carotid circulation. With hemodynamic transient ischemic attacks, emboli are not the cause of the cerebral dysfunction. More commonly, cardiac arrhythmias are associated with symptoms of global cerebral ischemia, i. e., lightheadedness, dizziness, giddiness, syncope, or convulsions. These global ischemic symptoms are most often seen in elderly patients.[11,12]

All patients with carotid transient ischemic attacks should have an electrocardiogram and a rhythm strip done, the latter being done at rest and after exercise. If any abnormality of rhythm is noted, the patient should have a Holter monitor to determine if the transient ischemic attacks are occurring when there is a change in the cardiac rhythm.[13,14] The physician must establish that the cardiac output does not play a primary role in the transient ischemic attacks before appropriate therapy can be instituted. The possibility that cardiac emboli can mimic transient ischemic attacks must always be considered. Here one must define a source for the cardiac emboli, i. e., those types of heart disease and heart arrhythmias that are often associated with embolic phenomena. In general, cardiac emboli produce symptoms which lead to the diagnosis of a completed stroke. However, if the emboli are small, the symptoms and signs can persist less than twenty-four hours and thus fall into the general classification of transient ischemic episodes.

In summary, the common symptoms of carotid transient ischemic attacks are:

1) monocular blindness or monocular blurring of vision in a previously normal eye

2) dysphasia (aphasic disorder)

3) contralateral weakness or numbness in the arm and leg individually or together

The following symptoms are <u>not</u> related to ischemia of the carotid artery system:

1) acute confusional states not representing aphasia

2) syncopal episodes

3) recurrent isolated headaches unassociated with other symptoms

4) convulsive seizures

5) scintillating scotoma

DIAGNOSTIC TESTS

Once the diagnosis of carotid transient ischemic attack is strongly considered, further studies are necessary to help substantiate this diagnosis.

Carotid bruits are vaguely discussed in the literature. The important characteristics of the bruits are its duration, pitch and loudness, and the presence or absence of an associated thrill on palpation. It is understood that cardiac murmurs can be transmitted to the carotid arteries in the neck; these must be differentiated from primary carotid bruits. In general, cardiac murmurs are loudest at their origin and decreased in intensity as they proceed distally.

A soft, high-pitched carotid bruit that spans systole and encroaches upon early diastole indicates a severe stenosis (greater than 85%) at the carotid bifurcation. A long medium-pitched coarse bruit spanning only systole, with or without a thrill, suggests significant irregularity in the intimal lining, and 50% or greater stenosis of the carotid lumen.

When feeling for thrills, please palpate gently at the carotid bifurcation and avoid stimulating the carotid sinus. Stimulation of the latter structure can often lead to severe bradycardia or cardiac arrest, particularly in older patients.

Short, medium or loud bruits that do not span systole can indicate narrowing, but one cannot draw any conclusions as to the degree of stenosis. Lastly, the presence of a carotid bruit is helpful in the diagnosis of carotid transient ischemic attacks, but the <u>absence</u> of a bruit does <u>not</u> rule out significant stenosis or an <u>ulcerated</u> plaque. Also, <u>one</u> should remember that carotid bruits sometimes occur from narrowing plaques in the proximal external carotid artery system.

Palpating the carotid artery to feel the magnitude of the systolic thrust is not useful in carotid disease. The carotid vessels vary in diameter and neck position. Even with total occlusion of the internal carotid artery, one cannot detect differences in the pulses, because on palpation the external carotid artery is felt. With common carotid artery occlusion, there is no pulse felt in the neck, and there is no pulse felt in the superficial temporal artery.

A bell-type stethoscope should be placed gently, lateral to the upper part of the thyroid cartilage and medial to the sternocleidomastoid muscle. From there it can be moved up slowly to the angle of the jaw. Sometimes one best hears bruits lower in the neck; but most often, the bruit is best heard at the angle of the jaw. When the bruit is heard, the physician should decrease the pressure on his stethoscope, because the pressure of the stethoscope on the carotid artery can produce an artefactual bruit. Auscultation should be done in a quiet room and the patient should be auscultated in both the sitting and supine positions, with the chin in a straight, anterior position. Occasionally, with total thrombosis of one internal carotid, a bruit is heard over the opposite carotid. This occurs because of increased blood flow through the uninvolved artery. A physiological hemodynamic-type bruit is also heard in some patients with anemia and in young children. High pitch bruits once heard with the bell-type stethoscope can often be better defined with a diaphragm scope.

There have been several noninvasive procedures devised to detect significant stenosis of the carotid artery system in the neck. None of these tests have been very useful in defining ulcerated nonstenotic plaques.[15]

Dynamic flow studies done with radioactive isotopes show flow through both carotid systems in the neck and intracranially. A significant delay in filling of the ipsilateral neck or the intracranial circulation is consistent with thrombosis or severe stenosis of the internal carotid artery. This test is crude at best and has proved to be of limited value even with total occlusion of the internal carotid artery system.

Carotid phonoangiography consists of audio-visual analysis of cervical carotid bruits. The equipment allows for more sophisticated evaluation of the bruit by the use of specially adapted microphones.[16] This technique is more accurate in evaluating the length and pitch of a carotid bruit.

Oculoplethysmography evaluates the transmission of pulse pressure via the ophthalmic artery and its retinal arterioles to the fluid medium of the globe. Abnormalities consist of delay in transmission, reduction in amplitude of the pulse wave, and variations in configuration of the pulse wave.

Oculoplethysmography can record the systolic arterial pressure in the eyes - comparing one side to another. A decrease of 33% or more indicates significant internal carotid stenosis on the ipsilateral side. A significant bilateral decrease in retinal artery pressure, compared to systemic arterial pressure, indicates bilateral carotid stenosis.

Both the procedures described require sophisticated equipment, plus physicians and technicians who are qualified to administer and evaluate the results. The literature suggests that both of these tests are capable of showing good correlation when the carotid artery stenosis is 50% or greater. However, as with all noninvasive procedures, there are false-positive and false-negative results.[17]

Doppler directional scanning has been developed to show reversal flow in the supra-orbital and trochlear branches of the ophthalmic artery. These arteries are branches from the internal carotid artery. The reversal flow in these vessels correlates well with a high degree of stenosis or total occlusion of the ipsilateral carotid artery.[18]

Facial thermography depicts decreased skin temperature in the facial areas supplied by the internal carotid artery. The decreased temperature suggests stenosis or occlusion of the ipsilateral internal carotid artery.[19] This test has rarely been used in recent years.

The ultrasound Doppler with the storage oscilloscope allows for imaging of the common carotid artery and its bifurcation in the neck; the imaging shows stenosis and occlusion in the internal carotid artery or in the common carotid artery. These procedures are said to have a 70 to 85% correlation when compared with carotid angiography. This test also requires sophisticated technicians and physicians to interpret the results.[20,21] More sophisticated equipment is now being produced. This procedure may well be the best for evaluating atherosclerotic carotid lesions. The essential use of these noninvasive procedures may be as a screening test for a given age population, who do not have symptoms and signs of transient ischemic attacks or strokes. Here, the tests may predict which asymptomatic patients are at risk for future ischemic or thrombotic lesions of the carotid system. These tests are also useful for following patients after carotid endarterection, i.e., local recurrence, thrombosis at surgery site, or progressive involvement of the opposite carotid artery.

The ultimate test for detecting intrinsic carotid disease is angiography.[22,23,24] This is usually done through the transfemoral route but can be done through the axillary route, or retrograde through the brachial artery. Direct carotid puncture is now used rarely for the diagnosis of atherosclerotic carotid disease.

When the physician finds it necessary to study the carotid artery and its branches in the neck, together with the intracranial circulation, it is best for the radiologist to place the catheter in the proximal lumen of the common carotid artery. Following the injection of contrast material, x-rays are taken in the AP, lateral and sometimes in the oblique positions. These x-rays will give good pictures of the common carotid artery, its bifurcation in the neck, and the intracranial circulation. When necessary, the catheter can then be placed in the opposite carotid artery and the procedure repeated. This type of study does not show the vertebral basilar system and does not show the proximal arteries that originate from the aortic arch.

With an aortic arch study, the catheter is placed in the aortic arch, and a large bolus of dye is injected. Following this injection, serial pictures are taken in at least two views which show the innominate artery at its take-off from the aortic arch and the bifurcation of the innominate artery into the common carotid and subclavian artery. The right common carotid artery and its bifurcation at the neck is also seen. On the left, the common carotid artery is seen at its take-off from the aortic arch, as well as the bifurcation of the common carotid artery in the neck. The physician is also able to see both subclavian arteries and the origin of the vertebral arteries from the subclavian arteries, plus the course of the vertebral arteries in the neck. The aortic arch studies do not show intracranial circulation; and in general, the delineation of the carotid system is not as clear as when catheterization of the vessels is done individually. The decision of what type of angiography is indicated will depend upon the patient's symptoms.

With the use of good subtraction films that remove bone from the picture and with magnification films, as well as good positioning, small ulcerated plaques in the posterior wall of the internal carotid artery can now be seen with ease. These angiographic procedures are now available in many hospitals. In addition, more radiology residents have been trained in neuroradiology, and they are capable of producing good studies. At the present time, the morbidity and mortality of angiography is quite low. An acceptable fixed neurologic morbidity rate should be between 0.5% and 1%. Mortality rates should not be greater than 0.1%.[25] As with all procedures, the adverse effects will depend on how often the procedure is done in your institution and on the skill and ability of the involved radiologist. If sophisticated neuroradiology is not available at your hospital, the patient should be transferred to more appropriate facilities.

Angiography should not be done in a patient with carotid transient ischemic attacks, unless the physician and the patient are willing to proceed with surgery when indicated. All patients should have good medical evaluations before proceeding with angiography. This should consist of a good history and physical examination, with careful attention to the heart, concerning angina, previous myocardial infarcts, congestive heart failure, murmurs, arrhythmias, and electrocardiogram abnormalities. Blood pressure should be recorded in both arms. The patient should be questioned about a history of hypertension or the use of antihypertensive medicines.

The abdomen should be examined for abdominal aneurysm and auscultated for any significant bruit. Careful history is to be taken concerning intermittent claudication with palpation and auscultation of the peripheral arteries. A chest x-ray is indicated for pulmonary disease, as well as cardiac size. An electrocardiogram should be done with a rhythm strip or Holter monitoring when indicated. Laboratory tests consist of CBC and differential, hematocrit, BUN, fasting blood sugar, and two-hour post-prandial sugar with glucose tolerance test, if indicated. Pulmonary function studies are necessary when indicated. Cholesterol and lipoprotein studies are indicated together with electrolytes.

A significant number of patients with carotid transient ischemic attacks have associated hypertension, diabetes mellitus, peripheral vascular disease, cardiac disease and hyperlipidemia. Rare cases are associated with polycythemia. The decision about therapy, in any given patient, cannot be intelligently made unless these associated disease processes are closely evaluated. It is important to understand that most patients with transient ischemic attacks eventually die from cardiac disease and not from stroke. Significant hypertension and diastolic pressures of 100 mm or greater of mercury increase the risk of cardiac disease, kidney disease, and cerebral hemorrhages.[26] Insulin-dependent diabetes mellitus of many years' duration produces diffuse premature atherosclerosis and increases the risk of both angiography and surgery. Significant cardiac disease, particularly congestive heart failure, increases the risk of angiography and surgery, plus it decreases the life expectancy of the patient.

THERAPY

Having made a clinical diagnosis of transient ischemic attacks of the carotid system, the physician must decide what further diagnoses or therapy are best for each particular patient. This simple statement belies the multiple complex and divergent approaches to the problem from both the medical and surgical standpoints. The literature is full of conflicting data. No one has all the correct answers. Common sense is important, as well as an open view of both the medical and surgical therapies. Selection of the appropriate therapy will also depend on the availability of radiological and surgical talent in your area. Surgical procedures should only be done in hospitals where many carotid vascular procedures are done each year. Chauvinism for one's institution is not acceptable if the risks increase the morbidity or the mortality to your patient.

The medical therapies available consist of platelet antagonists and Coumadin.[27, 28, 29] The term, platelet antagonist, has no precise meaning at this time; it has been used to describe drugs with any of the following properties. First, the drug can inhibit a measurable property of platelets, such as adhesion, retention, or aggregation when studies by in vivo techniques. Secondly, the drug can inhibit platelet-induced thrombus formation. Thirdly, it can prolong the survival of radioactively-labeled platelets in experimental or clinical conditions in which platelet survival is decreased. A drug might prolong platelet survival by suppressing platelet reactivity or by diminishing the underlying stimulus that has activated the platelet.[30] Individually, these drugs are:

1) Aspirin (acetylsalicylic acid)
2) Anturane (sulfinpyrazone)
3) Persantine (dipyridamole)
4) Coumadin (warfarin sodium)

Therapeutic doses for aspirin are 650 mg. b.i.d. or 325 mg. q.i.d.;* for Anturane, 200 mg. q.i.d., for Persantine, 200 to 400 mg./day; for Coumadin the prothrombin time should be kept at 2 to $2\frac{1}{2}$ times the normal control value.

In 1967, Weiss and Aledorf reported that platelet aggregation and release reaction were inhibited after ingestion of aspirin in man.[31] There is now considerable evidence that aspirin inhibits platelet aggregation and secretion by preventing the synthesis of prostaglandins and thromboxane A_2. It should be emphasized that aspirin only partially inhibits platelet aggregation. The inhibitory effect of aspirin on platelet aggregation, secretion and prostaglandin synthesis can be detected in the blood for four to seven days after ingestion of 325 mg. to 1300 mg. of the drug. There is no evidence that human platelets become refractory to the inhibitory effects of aspirin after long-term administration of large doses of the drug. Aspirin does not affect platelet survival, but it will prolong bleeding time.[32]

Anturane reduces platelet glass-adhesiveness and improves platelet survival, but it does not affect bleeding time in man, collagen-induced platelet aggregation, or the release reaction. It has been suggested that Anturane acts on the vessel wall rather than on the platelets themselves. At present, Anturane is used as a uricosuric agent in the treatment of gout. Recent studies have suggested that Anturane might decrease the mortality from myocardial infarcts in patients being treated

---

* Recent in vivo studies suggest that the dose of aspirin necessary to coat platelets, may be much less than noted above.

with this medication for gout and in patients with a previous history of a myocardial infarct.[33]

Persantine was introduced as a coronary vasodilator in 1961. The antithrombotic properties of the drug were reported in 1965 by Emons, et al. who showed that the drug inhibited platelet-induced thromboembolism in the cerebrocortical blood vessels of rabbits.[34] Similar results have been obtained in other experimental models.[35] At present, it is not clear how Persantine inhibits platelet-induced thrombosis in man.

Fields and his colleagues have recently reported a controlled clinical trial of aspirin for treatment of cerebral ischemia.[36] Patients who have had transient ischemic attacks in the carotid artery distribution were randomly assigned to aspirin or to a placebo. They were followed to determine the incidences of subsequent transient ischemic attacks, retinal infarctions, cerebral infarctions, and death. The six-month follow-up to date shows substantial differential in favor of aspirin. Indication in favor of aspirin treatment was primarily in persons with a history of numerous carotid transient ischemic attacks and in patients whose symptoms were likely to have resulted from angiographically demonstrable carotid lesions.

The recent Canadian cooperative study on aspirin and sulfinpyrazone is by far the best controlled study to date.[37] It indicates unequivocally that aspirin is beneficial in reducing the risks of transient ischemic attacks, strokes, and death in patients with a previous history of occlusive vascular disease. The dosage of aspirin was 325 mg. q.i.d. Aspirin produced a risk reduction of 19% for continuing transient attacks, stroke, or death. For more clinically important events, such as stroke or death, the risk reduction was 31%. Aspirin was effective in diabetic patients but was not as nearly effective in patients with a previous history of a myocardial infarct.

The response in women on aspirin therapy was disappointing. There was no statistical evidence that aspirin reduced the incidence of transient ischemic attacks, stroke, or death in the female.

Sulfinpyrazone did not produce a statistically significant risk reduction in any of the categories.

More controlled studies will be necessary in the future. For the present, aspirin should be recommended on a long-term basis for all males with carotid transient ischemic attacks or completed stroke that do not have surgically removable lesions. It should also be used on a long-term basis in all male patients after carotid endarterectomy. Despite the relatively poor effects on male patients with previous myocardial infarction, aspirin should still be prescribed. On the dosage schedule previously noted, there were very few gastrointestinal side effects when aspirin was given alone.

In women, aspirin therapy will be speculative until further controlled studies are completed. Since there is little evidence of beneficial effects from Persantine in occlusive vascular disease, and since sulfinpyrazone appears ineffective, we should continue with aspirin therapy until further studies prove or disprove the sex-dependent difference.

Long-term therapy with Coumadin provides the following data: Therapy is effective in decreasing or stopping carotid transient ischemic attacks but does not decrease subsequent cerebral thrombosis or death.[38] In addition, it is difficult to keep the prothrombin time at a therapeutic level unless the patient is very cooperative and intelligent. Furthermore, there are significant bleeding complications more in elderly patients, even in the best controlled studies.[39]

The use of Coumadin in medically treated transient ischemic attacks should be reserved for only those patients who do not respond to platelet antagonists. In addition, Coumadin therapy should be limited to three to six months; then the medication should be stopped to see if the transient ischemic attacks will recur. Sometimes, transient ischemic attacks will stop spontaneously.

The primary therapeutic problem is to decide which cases will be treated medically, which cases will have angiography, and ultimately, which cases will be selected for surgery.

In 1954, Carrea and his colleagues in Buenos Aires reported the first successful extradural carotid artery reconstruction which had previously been performed in 1951. Since then there have been dramatic advances in all phases of this surgery. The operative mortality for carotid surgery on patients with transient ischemic attacks is about 0.8% in sophisticated centers. Morbidity consists of 0.9% transient deficit and 0.7% permanent neurological deficits.[40, 41, 42, 43, 44]

Most sophisticated vascular surgeons use an internal shunt with endarterectomy. This allows for continued perfusion of the carotid circulation during the procedure, giving the surgeon adequate time to remove the atherosclerotic plaque in toto. Other vascular surgeons do not use an internal shunt unless there is no back pressure present when the carotid vessel is totally occluded at the time of the surgery.[45]

Some of the procedures are done under local anesthesia and others under general anesthesia. Some surgeons use hypoventilation, some use hyperventilation, and some artifically raise the blood pressure during surgery. All of these modifications are done in order to improve cerebral blood flow and protect the brain against ischemia and infarction.

The type and duration of the ischemic symptoms play a significant role in determining the appropriate therapy. Patients with <u>frequent</u> transient ischemic attacks of the internal carotid artery system should be anticoagulated with heparin, until the attacks stop completely; these patients are a high risk to develop a completed stroke. Angiography should be done as soon as possible.

One attack of amaurosis fugax can easily be treated with aspirin. However, it is probably better to study the involved carotid vessel first, in any patient who is a good surgical candidate. The arteriogram should <u>only</u> be done if the physician is convinced that the diagnosis of amaurosis fugax is definitive. If the physician chooses to use anti-platelet therapy, then angiography can be carried out if the patient develops recurrent attacks of amaurosis fugax, despite this therapy. The presence of a significant bruit or thrill in a patient with amaurosis fugax is unequivocal evidence that the patient should have angiography to delineate the size and the position of the lesion. If the angiography demonstrates marked stenosis (greater than 50%), surgery should be performed. At the time of the initial carotid angiogram, the opposite carotid system must be studied if there is any significant pathology present on the symptomatic side. The surgeon should not operate on any carotid artery unless he is aware of the patency of the opposite carotid artery and the intracranial circulation. Today, most vascular surgeons, neurosurgeons and neurologists would consider an ulcerating plaque, with or without stenosis, as a definite indication for carotid surgery if the patient has symptoms in the involved carotid circulation.[46]

Often the patient with amaurosis fugax has total occlusion of the ipsilateral carotid artery. In this situation, the opposite carotid artery should be studied. If there is a significant lesion in the opposite carotid vessel, consisting of a high degree of stenosis, then surgery on the noninvolved side would appear indicated. If the patient has only an ulcerated plaque or a small degree of stenosis in the opposite asymptomatic carotid artery, he or she should be treated with aspirin and followed. Surgery is not indicated at that time. If, despite the anti-platelet therapy, the patient goes on to develop symptoms or signs indicating progressive disease of the opposite carotid system, then surgery can be performed on the involved vessel at that time.

In some patients with amaurosis fugax, the study of the involved carotid artery system will be negative. In these patients, the emboli may be coming proximally from the carotid artery or the aortic arch on the involved side. These patients should be treated with long-term aspirin in an attempt to control the visual symptoms. If the aspirin fails, the patient is entitled to a course of Coumadin therapy as previously described.

All patients with ischemic carotid symptoms that last for hours or longer, particularly those with aphasia, should have angiography, even if all noninvasive studies are negative, including the absence of bruits. The damaging effect of permanent aphasia or hemiplegias cannot be overemphasized.

Patients with multiple brief carotid transient ischemic episodes that produce weakness or numbness of the opposite extremities, should be studied by angiography as soon as the physician is secure about the diagnosis.

Recent microvascular surgery, with anastomoses of the superficial temporal artery to a branch of the middle cerebral artery, has been carried out in patients with total occlusion of the internal carotid artery and persistent transient ischemic attacks in the same circulation. To date, the effectiveness of the above procedure is not known.

Patients presenting with asymptomatic carotid bruits should be evaluated carefully.[47] If the bruit is loud and extends through systole with or without an associated thrill, carotid angiography is indicated. If noninvasive studies demonstrate significant stenosis, carotid angiogram is also indicated. If the stenosis of the involved side is 50% or greater and ulcerated, the atherosclerotic plaque should be removed. It must be remembered that atherosclerosis is a progressive disease. If the plaque is not removed, it may become larger, and with time, the patient may develop either transient ischemic attacks from micro-emboli or go on to total occlusion of the involved internal carotid artery. It is an axiom that all patients are better off when both carotid arteries are patent.

The surgical statistics quoted previously will be less impressive in different areas of the country where the sophistication and experience are less. The mortality and morbility of surgery will be higher in patients with advanced atherosclerotic heart disease, congestive heart failure, obesity, significant long-standing diabetes mellitus, and uncontrolled essential hypertension, as well as in patients over the age of seventy. In addition, in patients who have transient ischemic attacks of both the vertebral basilar and the carotid system, the surgical morbidity is higher than the original figures quoted.

Be very cautious about recommending angiographic studies for carotid disease in patients with pre-senile or senile dementia. These disease processes are not due to cerebral ischemia but reflect premature degeneration of the cortical cells.

The patient that is demented, secondary to severe bilateral carotid stenosis, is a very rare entity. There are some patients with dementia due to occlusive vascular disease of the cerebrum. A good history and neurological examination will indicate the presence of multiple previous strokes[48] (Multi-infarct dementia).

There is no indication for entertaining the diagnosis of carotid artery ischemia in patients with isolated ipsilateral headaches, syncopal episodes, confusional states, or convulsions.

In summary, consult both a neurologist and a vascular surgeon in each case. Use your medical judgement and knowledge of the patient to help with an appropriate decision. Be judicious and thoughtful and remember that you can't make the right decision every time.[49]

If the neurologist and the vascular surgeon disagree, the final decision should be made by you and your patient after you have given the patient a summary of both consulting views.

PART TWO: VERTEBRAL BASILAR SYSTEM

GENERAL INFORMATION

There are divergent thoughts concerning the etiology of ischemic episodes in the vertebral basilar system. Some involved specialists feel that they are secondary to platelet-fibrin or atherosclerotic emboli, and others feel that the ischemic episodes are related to a decrease in the total blood flow through the posterior circulation. The probable truth is that both types are involved in different episodes; however, no one knows which form predominates. Unlike the carotid-retinal circulation, emboli cannot be seen in the vertebral basilar artery system. The difficulty in determining the specific etiology for any given episode probably is the cause of the conflicting data and reports concerning therapeutic results in this type of disease process.

The vertebral arteries arise from the subclavian arteries and course lateral to the vertebral bodies, entering the skull through the foramen magnum. At the medullary pontine junction, the vertebral arteries join to form the basilar artery. The basilar artery runs along the ventral part of the brain stem until it terminates into two posterior cerebral arteries. The vertebral basilar artery system supplies the brain stem, the cerebellum, the thalmus, the occipital lobes, and medial inferior temporal lobes. The communication between the anterior circulation and the posterior circulation is carried out through the posterior communicating artery; this is a branch from the internal carotid artery that anastomoses with the posterior cerebral artery completing the circle of Willis. In the brain stem, the vertebral basilar circulation gives off multiple lateral and median penetrating arteries that supply all structures in the posterior fossa.

Atherosclerotic plaquing in the vertebral basilar system is more diffuse than that noted in the carotid system. While there is a definitive plaquing seen at the junction of the vertebral take-off from the subclavian arteries, there is also multiple plaquing throughout the course of the entire system. This clearly explains why surgery at the subclavian vertebral junction has been unproductive through the years, in relieving symptoms of vertebral basilar transient ischemic attacks.[50]

One vertebral artery is most often larger than the other, with the left being the predominating vessel. In some cases, almost the entire blood supply of the vertebral basilar system will come from one vertebral artery.

The diagnosis of transient ischemic attacks in the vertebral basilar system is more difficult than the transient ischemic attacks that involve the carotid system. The common presenting symptoms are bilateral visual blurring, diplopia, ataxia, and drop spells.[9] Bilateral motor and sensory changes are rare; but when they occur, they clearly reflect ischemia in the posterior circulation. Numbness involving both sides of the face, both sides of the tongue and/or mouth, is unequivocal evidence of vertebral basilar disease. Motor or sensory changes that involve different sides during different attacks are also indicative of vertebral basilar disease, as are crossed syndromes that involve one side of the face and the opposite extremities.

For an accurate diagnosis of transient ischemic attacks of the vertebral basilar system, one should always look for a combination of the symptoms previously noted. It will be very difficult to make a diagnosis on the basis of the single attack with an isolated symptom.[8] Even with repetitive attacks producing one symptom, the physician must be careful before drawing any definite conclusions. As with carotid disease, the physician can increase his accuracy greatly if he is present during the attack, i.e., the presence of nystagmus, cerebellar ataxia, paresis of the extraocular muscles, bilateral Babinski signs, bilateral motor weakness, bilateral sensory deficit, bilateral visual loss, and crossed syndromes. In addition, evaluation of the state of consciousness and the cardiac system at the time of the attack will be helpful.

DIFFERENTIAL DIAGNOSIS

Recurrent episodes of true vertigo occur with transient ischemic attacks of the vertebral basilar system. Do not accept lightheadedness, wooziness, giddiness, or nonspecific symptoms of dizziness. Vertigo entails true spinning of the environment, or of the patient. Recurrent vertigo also occurs with Meniere's disease. The latter disease is usually present in a younger age group and is almost always associated with significant unilateral or bilateral hearing loss. Be very careful to exclude all dizzy episodes that occur with postural changes. In addition, be cautious about dizziness which is an isolated symptom secondary to generalized decrease in cerebral blood flow from a cardiac arrhythmia.

Intermittent diplopia can be caused by increased intracranial pressure, myasthenia gravis, and endocrine abnormality such as Graves' disease. Always ask the patient to close one eye in order to determine if the diplopia disappears. Monocular diplopia is very rarely a symptom of organic central nervous system disease. Some patients only have diplopia in certain directions of gaze, and this may be confused with intermittent diplopia. In these patients, a careful red glass test done by an ophthalmologist may show the presence of a permanent weakness in one of the extraocular muscles which would exclude the diagnosis of transient ischemic attacks of the vertebral basilar system.

Bilateral visual blurring in vertebral basilar ischemia is often described as a curtain coming down over both eyes. However, patients with syncope related to decreased cardiac output often complain of blurred vision or "graying out", prior to losing consciousness. Unless the patient is crystal clear throughout the attack and can give a good history, one must be very careful in making a diagnosis of transient ischemic attacks rather than generalized cerebral ischemia on the basis of blurred vision alone.

Episodic ataxia is seen with the use of alcohol and several drugs. In addition, patients with Parkinson's disease and associated gait problems are often thought to have ataxia because they fall a great deal. A good history and physical examination will clearly exclude the patients whose ataxia is due to Parkinson's disease.

Drop spells are described as a sudden loss of strength or tone in the lower extremities that cause the patient to fall to the ground with no loss of consciousness. The patient is usually able to get up and walk around within minutes and must be completely clear during the episodes. However, as described previously, elderly patients can fall down from Parkinson's disease; they also can fall when suffering from carotid sinus hypersensitivity or cardiac arrhythmias. It is important to document palpitations, turning of the neck quickly to one side or the other, or touching the neck in the area close to the carotid sinus, prior to the falling. Older patients often have difficulty with recent memory and recall; and in addition, they are frightened by these episodes. All of these factors add up to decreasing the accuracy when using the history alone to make a correct diagnosis. The physician will have to be patient before coming to a definite conclusion about diagnosis of ischemia in the posterior circulation. As alluded to before, careful attention must be given to the cardiac status in each patient to rule out the possibility that the central nervous system symptoms are not related to a significant decrease in cardiac output. If a spouse or a relative is near the patient during an attack, this may be very helpful in getting a more accurate history.

As with carotid transient ischemic attacks, all symptoms and signs in vertebral basilar ischemia must be gone by twenty-four hours. If the symptoms and signs persist longer, they cannot be classified as transient ischemic attacks. Persistent posterior fossa signs must be studied carefully to differentiate completed stroke from other diseases in that area. Combinations of two or more symptoms previously described such as bilateral visual blurring, true vertigo, ataxia, drop spells, bilateral motor or sensory changes or crossed syndromes will help immensely in making an accurate diagnosis.

The vertebral basilar form of migraine closely mimics transient ischemic attacks of the vertebral basilar system. The patient is generally in a younger age group and the attacks are often followed by significant headaches. There is often a family history of recurrent migraine attacks. The symptoms of vertebral basilar ischemia are identical to those reported with vertebral basilar migraine, with the exception that the motor and sensory symptoms often have a spreading or marching quality in the latter disease.

Transient global amnesia is not accepted by most neurologists as a symptom complex related to vertebral basilar ischemia. The patient is usually over the age of fifty. He has a sudden onset of recent memory disturbance; he is not able to record what is taking place during the attack; he asks repetitive questions despite being given adequate answers; he is confused and anxious during the attack. The attack may last from several hours to most of a day. The symptoms disappear rapidly and it is apparent the patient has very significant amnesia for what went on during the episode. It is uncommon for these episodes to recur. When the patient is seen during an attack, it is easy to determine that he is not recording recent events by giving him several names and asking him to repeat them minutes later. He will be unable to retain what was given to him, even if he is questioned shortly after the information has been given. There are some neurologists who feel there is often evidence of diffuse atherosclerosis or hypertension in this type of patient, and these neurologists are the ones who feel that this may represent a vascular ischemic episode. They postulate that the patient is having decreased blood flow to the medial temporal lobes, and these structures are those that are involved in retention of recent memory. Since the medial temporal lobes are supplied by the vertebral basilar system, the feeling is that the ischemia is along those arteries. This entity should be recognized as not of psychiatric origin, but at this time should not be placed under the classification of transient ischemic attacks of the vertebral basilar system.[51]

Auscultation above the middle of the clavicle may reveal a bruit, suggesting stenosis at the subclavian-vertebral junction. However, in some classic cases of transient ischemic attacks of the vertebral basilar system, there are significant associated unilateral or bilateral carotid bruits. The bruit is less important than the symptoms and signs when determining which system is involved. In certain cases noted previously, the patient can have transient ischemic attacks involving both systems.

Unlike the carotid artery system, we do not have useful noninvasive tests to delineate significant narrowing in the vertebral basilar artery system. Dynamic radioactive isotope studies have been used, but the results, in general, have been disappointing in delineating occlusion or narrowing of the vertebral arteries.

In each patient with transient ischemic attacks of the vertebral basilar system, the physician must look for stenosis of other vessels that could lead to these symptoms, i.e., occlusion or significant narrowing of the innominate artery, occlusion or stenosis of the subclavian arteries proximal to the take-off of the vertebral arteries. Medium and high-pitched, long bruits or thrills over the subclavian arteries, pulse delays in one or the other radial artery at the wrist, and significant differences of blood pressure in the two arms will all be helpful.

A great deal has been written in medical literature about the subclavian steal.[52] This is a very rare clinical entity. In the classic form, the patient should develop symptoms and signs of vertebral basilar ischemia with active exercise of one arm. On the left, this would occur because of stenosis of the subclavian artery proximal to the vertebral take-off. With exercise of the left arm and ischemia, the vertebral artery blood flow reverses and supplies blood to the left arm. On the right, this can occur with either innominate artery disease or subclavian disease; again, there is a reversal of flow to increase the blood supply to the ischemic right arm. Usefulness of this syndrome is to document the fact that there are hemodynamic transient ischemic attacks of the vertebral basilar system.

On rare occasions, the patients can get classic symptoms of vertebral basilar ischemia when they turn their neck to one side or the other. This may be due to a large lateral osteoarthritic spur which compresses the main vertebral artery when the spur is placed in opposition to that artery. In most of these patients, the opposite vertebral artery is very small, hypoplastic, or totally thrombosed.

THERAPY

Previously, most aortic arch studies done for posterior circulation disease were carried out to delineate abnormalities at the subclavian vertebral junction. With time, it has become apparent that the arch studies are indicated primarily for posterior circulation patients that have disease processes in the large vessels, such as the innominate artery or the subclavian arteries.[23] Arteriograms are important in these patients because surgery has been useful in removing the stenosis or in bypassing the stenosis by arterial grafts. There is a good consensus of opinion that if surgery is indicated in vertebral basilar transient ischemic attacks, it is indicated for those persons with major vessel disease proximal to the take-off of the subclavian vertebral junction.[46]

However, the majority of patients with transient ischemic attacks of the vertebral basilar system do not have significant stenosis in the major vessels. Surgery directed towards improving the stenosis or ulceration at the subclavian vertebral junction has been universally disappointing through the years. There seems little question that this is because of the diffuse atherosclerosis involving multiple areas in the vertebral basilar system. In the absence of abnormalities noted in the large vessels described previously, an aortic arch study is no longer necessary to confirm the diagnosis of vertebral basilar ischemia.

Some patients with classic vertebral basilar ischemia have loud bruits over one or both carotid arteries. There are some surgeons who feel that in these particular patients it is important to remove significant stenosis from the carotid arteries. They feel that improvement of the cerebral blood flow through the carotid vessels will increase the blood flow to the posterior circulation via both posterior communicating arteries. The data concerning this type of surgery are very conflicting. There are some reports of significant decrease in vertebral basilar transient ischemic attacks after unilateral or bilateral carotid endarterectomies.[53] There are other reports indicating absolutely no improvement from carotid surgery.[54] It is apparent that the carotid surgery will not be effective unless the patient has very significant stenosis (95 to 99%) in one or both carotid vessels, and unless the posterior communicating arteries are patent; embolic episodes in the vertebral basilar system are never going to be helped by any type of carotid surgery. In addition, removal of nonstenotic ulcerated plaques from the carotid system are not going to help patients with vertebral basilar ischemia. The conflicting reports may be related to the fact that we have both a hemodynamic etiology and a thrombo-emboli etiology. Improving the flow to the anterior circulation might help in the former, but certainly does not help in the latter.

There is almost universal agreement that in most cases of transient ischemic attacks of the vertebral basilar system the treatment of choice should be to use the anti-platelet medication.[28] One should use aspirin at a dose of 650 mg. b.i.d. or 325 mg. q.i.d. This medication should be continued on a long-term basis for all patients with transient ischemic attacks or completed strokes involving the vertebral basilar system. Since this is a relatively benign form of therapy, it can be started in some patients even if the diagnosis of vertebral basilar ischemia is not made with any certainty. The goal of therapy will be to stop or greatly decrease the number of transient ischemic attacks and to prevent a completed stroke or death. In the cases where anti-platelet medication does not stop the transient ischemic attacks, a course of Coumadin therapy is indicated, as described previously. The latter drug should be used only for those patients who are not responding at all to the anti-platelet drugs and only for those patients who have had frequent enough transient ischemic attacks of the posterior circulation to interfere with their normal living. As stressed previously, Coumadin should not be used in older patients with dementia or in uncooperative patients, or in patients who are prone to falling.

The use of vasodilator drugs has been disappointing in treating patients with transient ischemic attacks. Despite the fact that some vasodilators increase the cerebral blood flow, there has been no convincing evidence that they are of any value in patients with transient ischemic attacks.[55]

In all patients, careful attention is to be directed toward keeping the cardiac output at an optimal level and preventing or treating cardiac arrhythmias that might be precipitating transient ischemic episodes. The physician should also pay careful attention to controlling hypertension, diabetes mellitus, and hyperlipidemia. Obese patients should be placed on appropriate diets; and exercise programs for all groups of patients are certainly indicated, when possible, to improve cardiac function. Patients with polycythemia or other hyperviscosity syndromes should have appropriate medical treatment. Dehydration is to be avoided in all of these patients because of its obvious detrimental effects in circulatory problems. Needless to say, the adverse effects of cigarette smoking in all patients with circulatory diseases should be stressed.

In distinction to transient ischemic attacks of the carotid artery system, patients with transient ischemic attacks of the vertebral basilar system will be primarily cared for by the internist or primary physician. These physicians will be responsible for a holistic approach to the patient, i.e., giving patient total care for all those disease processes which can aggravate transient ischemic attacks and lead to premature atherosclerosis.

The primary physician will make the best judgements by handling each case on an individual basis. The physician can use whatever form of therapy he thinks is most appropriate for the individual patient. The primary physician is the best judge as to which form or forms of therapy will be best tolerated by and most acceptable to the patient, so that therapy will be carried out consistently.

Until we determine the specific cause for atherosclerosis and develop a specific treatment, the physician will have to use the methods described in the previous chapter with the total understanding that these forms of therapy are less than optimal.

CASE STUDIES

CASE 1:

This 50-year-old right-handed, white female housewife was admitted to the hospital.

Four weeks prior to admission, while working in the kitchen, she had a sudden onset of a left frontal headache. She dropped a spoon out of her right hand, and when she bent over to pick it up, she could not get it with her right hand. She was not sure whether the hand was clumsy or weak. The hand improved in a few minutes. There was no leg weakness, aphasia, paresthesias, or loss of vision. About the same time, she noted a "whooshing" sound in her left temple that coincided with her pulse. The sound has persisted to the present.

Since then, she has had three or four more similar episodes of difficulty using the right arm; they all resolved without residual deficit. She has also had one episode when, "I knew what I wanted to say but couldn't get it out." This lasted a few minutes and was not accompanied by weakness.

She saw her local physician; brain scan and skull series were normal; she has had high blood pressure for years, controlled on diuretics. No diabetes, or family history of stroke.

PHYSICIAN EXAMINATION:

BP: 140/80 in both arms; Pulse: 80, regular; T: 98.6 degrees F; R: 16. General physical examination was unremarkable. No skin rash. No heart murmur. Neurological exam revealed her to be alert and oriented x 3. Language function and memory were good. There was good muscle power throughout. Sensory and cerebellar examinations were unremarkable. Cranial nerves were intact except for a left Horner's syndrome, without anhydrosis. Reflexes were symmetrical and plantar responses flexor bilaterally. There was a soft, short bruit over the bifurcation of the left carotid. Short, systolic bruits were also heard over both temples and both eyes. These bruits disappeared with left common carotid compression.

LABORATORY DATA:

CBC; urinalysis; platelet count; Sed. rate; SMA-12 (Blood sugar, BUN, creatinine, uric acid, cholesterol, CO_2, chlorides, sodium, potassium, alkaline phosphatase, SGOT); EKG; CFS; triglycerides; and chest x-ray were all normal.

We felt that she was having multiple transient ischemic attacks of the left internal carotid artery system. The unusual feature was the intracranial bruits and the patient's awareness of the noise over the left side of her head.

Bilateral carotid angiography, via femoral catheter, revealed 25% stenosis with post-stenotic dilation of the proximal internal carotid artery at its origin from the right common carotid artery. A similar defect was seen on the left. In addition, she had severe narrowing of the left internal carotid artery throughout its course in the Petrous bone. The vessel was one-third normal size. There were several plaques seen in the stenotic area.

The stenotic plaque at the carotid bifurcation on the left could be surgically removed, but we felt that the bruit and the transient ischemic attacks were arising from the stenotic internal carotid artery in the Petrous bone. This area was not surgically approachable. The patient was discharged on 325mg of aspirin twice a day. She will be followed closely for further transient ischemic attacks. We plan to readmit her to the hospital in about six months to repeat the left carotid angiogram. If she develops a total occlusion of the left internal carotid artery in the Petrous bone, she will be a surgical candidate for a superficial temporal artery-middle cerebral artery system bypass. This procedure is now in its experimental phase with the hope that it will improve collateral blood flow to the middle cerebral artery system.

CASE 2:

A 67-year-old, white female was admitted to the hospital because of repetitive attacks of short duration (1-2 minutes), characterized by true vertigo, diplopia and numbness in all extremities. In the past four months, she had a total of sixteen attacks. She is known to have had diabetes mellitus for ten years and uses oral medication and diet. There is no history of hypertension, heart disease or intermittent claudication.

The patient was alert, oriented without dementia. Neurological examination was essentially negative. Blood pressure was 130/70 in the right arm and 140/80 in the left arm. The general physical examination was unremarkable.

She had a loud, short bruit over the right subclavian artery associated with a thrill. No other bruits were present.

CBC, urinalysis, chest x-ray, EKG, were normal. SMA-12 was normal except for a blood sugar of 200 mg.% and cholesterol of 320 mg.%.

We felt that the patient had transient ischemic attacks involving the vertebral basilar system. The possibility existed that she had a thrombosed or atrophic left vertebral artery, associated with significant stenosis of the subclavian artery on the right proximal to the vertebral origin. Under these circumstances, surgery to remove the subclavian stenosis could help improve circulation through the right vertebral artery.

An aortic arch study was done, via femoral catheter. This revealed total occlusion of the left internal carotid artery. The left vertebral artery was of normal size and free of plaques.

There was a 25% narrowing and irregularity of the intima in the proximal subclavian artery on the right. The right internal carotid artery was 25% stenotic at its origin from the common carotid artery. The innominate artery showed multiple plaquing. The right vertebral artery was normal in size and showed a small plaque at its origin.

This patient was not a candidate for surgery. She was discharged on 325 mg. of aspirin b.i.d.

If the ischemic attacks continue to recur frequently in the future despite the aspirin, we will then initiate a course of Coumadin therapy. This patient is intelligent, reliable and can be followed closely.

::

CASE 3:

A seventy-two-year-old white male was admitted to the surgical service of the hospital. He had been bothered with intermittent claudication for six months and complained that the pain in his calves was becoming more severe with time. He could now only walk about one block before the onset of pain and would have to stop and rest until the pain disappeared. The patient has had diabetes mellitus for ten years and took Diabenase two per day and followed a diet. He was known to be normotensive with a blood pressure of 130/80; his electrocardiogram taken previously showed flattened T-waves in V-5 and V-6, but otherwise it was within normal limits. SMA-12 was normal except for a blood sugar of 180 mg.% and a serum cholesterol of 320 mg.%. CBC and urinalysis were normal. Chest x-ray was normal.

The patient had been previously admitted to the hospital where arteriography was done, and it was felt that he required bilateral iliofemoral bypasses. At the time of admission, the neurological examination revealed a loud, short bruit over the right carotid artery at the angle of the jaw and a very long loud bruit over the left internal carotid artery at the angle of the jaw; the latter was associated with a thrill on palpation. There was a very short soft bruit above the middle of the right clavicle. The remainder of the neurological examination was completely within normal limits. A careful history failed to reveal any previous symptoms to suggest transient ischemic attacks of the carotid or vertebral basilar artery system.

On the advice of the neurological service, bilateral carotid angiography was carried out via the femoral route despite the local vascular disease in the femoral arteries. The right internal carotid artery was narrowed about 50% just distal to the carotid bifurcation. There was no ulceration noted on the stenotic plaque. There was 90% or greater narrowing of the left internal carotid artery distal to the bifurcation on the left. There was definite irregularity on the intimal surface of the stenotic plaque on the left. There was a slight stenotic plaque at the origin of the right vertebral artery from the subclavian artery but no other gross abnormalities were noted. The intracranial circulation, particularly of the middle and the anterior cerebral artery systems, was normal bilaterally.

The vascular service was advised to perform a carotid endarterectomy on the left prior to carrying out iliofemoral bypasses. We felt that there was a significant narrowing on the left which could precipitate a completed stroke of the left internal carotid artery system if the patient's blood pressure dropped at the time of the abdominal surgery. Subsequently, the atherosclerotic plaque was removed from the left internal carotid artery via an internal shunt. There was definite ulceration and irregularity of the intimal surface. The patient tolerated the procedure well. Two weeks later the femoral bypasses were done. The patient tolerated these procedures well. He was discharged on aspirin 650 mg. twice a day.

If the carotid angiography revealed a stenotic lesion of 50% or less, we would not have recommended that carotid surgery be carried out prophylactically. Thrombo-embolic complications from ulcerated lesions are not more prone to occur during periods of hypotension. However, in the presence of a significant stenosis a drop in the blood pressure could be quite crucial to the involved cerebral circulation.

This case illustrates the need to individualize. Prophylactic carotid surgery is <u>not</u> needed in every patient prior to abdominal or peripheral vascular surgery, unless vascular studies reveal significant stenosis that may lead to a completed stroke in the event of a drop in blood pressure.

::

REFERENCES

1. J.P. Whisnant, et al.: Transient Cerebral Ischemic Attacks in a Community; Rochester, Minnesota, 1955 - 1969. Mayo Clinic Proc. 48:194, 1973.

2. H. Eisenberg, J.T. Morrison, et al: Cerebrovascular Accidents; Incidence and Survival Rates in a Defined Population, Middlesex County, Connecticut. JAMA 189:883, 1964.

3. W.S. Fields, V. Maslenikov, et al.: Joint Study of Extracranial Arterial Occlusion V Report of Prognosis Following Surgery or Nonsurgical Treatment for Transient Cerebral Ischemic Attack and Cervical Carotid Artery Lesions. JAMA 211:1993, March 23, 1970.

4. R.N. McClelland, Editor: Selected Readings in General Surgery. Cerebrovascular Disease, Vol. III, Number 11, November, 1976.

5. W.S. Fields and N.A. Lemak: Joint Study of Extracranial Arterial Occlusion, X Internal Carotid Artery Occlusion. JAMA 235:2734, 1976.

6. A. Heyman, et al.: XI Transient Focal Cerebral Ischemia: Epidemiological and Clinical Aspects. Stroke 5:277, 1974.

7. T.R. Price, et al.: Cooperative Study of Hospital Frequency and Character of Transient Ischemic Attacks, VI Patients Examined During an Attack. JAMA 238:2512, 1977.

8. P.R. Calanchini, et al.: Cooperative Study of Hospital Frequency and Character of Transient Ischemic Attacks, The Reliability of Diagnosis. JAMA 238:2029, 1977.

9. D.E. Futty, et al.: Cooperative Study of Hospital Frequency and Character of Transient Ischemic Attacks, Symptom Analysis. JAMA 238:2386, 1977.

10. J.F. Toole, R. Janeway, et al.: Transient Ischemic Attacks Due to Atherosclerosis Prospective Study of 160 Patients. Archives of Neurology 32:5, 1975.

11. Robert L. Reed, Robert Siekert, et al.: Rarity of Transient Focal Cerebral Ischemia in Cardiac Dysrhythmia. JAMA 223:893, 1973.

12. J.P. Van Durme: Tachyarrhythmias and Transient Cerebral Ischemic Attacks. American Heart Journal 89:538, 1975.

13. J. Sterlin, I. Klein, et al.: Importance of Holter Monitoring in Patients with Periodic Cerebral Symptoms. Annals of Neurology 1:470, May, 1977.

14. N.J. Holter: New Methods for Heart Studies. Science 134:1214, 1961.

15. G.E. Bone, and R.W. Barnes: Limitations of the Doppler Cerebrovascular Examination in Hemispheric Cerebral Ischemia. Surgery 79:577, May, 1976.

16. M.M. Kartchner, et al.: Non-Invasive Detection and Evaluation of Carotid Occlusive Disease. Archives of Surgery 106:528, 1973.

17. B.J. Sand, et al.: Ophthalmic Arterial Blood Pressures Measured by Ocular Plethysmdynamography. Archives of Surgery 110:813, 1975.

18. D. Katz, R. Smith, et al.: Doppler Sonography Diagnosis of Cerebrovascular Disease. Stroke 7:439, 1976.

19. T.D. Capistrant: Thermographic Facial Patterns in Carotid Occlusive Disease. Radiology 100:85, July, 1971.

20. R.W. Barnes, et al.: Non-Invasive Ultrasound Carotid Angiography: Prospective Validation by Contrast Arteriography. Surgery 80:328, September, 1976.

21. E. Blackwell, J. Merary, et al.: Doppler Ultrasound Scanning of the Carotid Bifurcation. Archives of Neurology 34:145, 1977.

22. P.D. Swanson, et al.: Cooperative Study of Hospital Frequency and Character of Transient Ischemic Attacks, II Performance of Angiography Among Six Centers. JAMA 237:2202, 1977.

23. W.K. Hass, W.S. Fields, et al.: Joint Study of Extracranial Arterial Occlusion, II Arteriography, Techniques, Sites, and Complications. JAMA 203:961, 1968.

24. J.S. Pessin, G.W. Duncan, et al.: Clinical and Angiographic Features of Carotid Transient Ischemic Attacks. New England Journal of Medicine 296:358, 1977.

25. R.L. Mani: Review of Complications of Femorocerebral Catheter Angiography, Diagnostic Radiology, 1976, Margulis and Gooding, eds., pp. 797-812.

26. Editorial: Effect of Antihypertensive Treatment on Stroke Recurrence. JAMA 229:409, 1974.

27. F.M. Yatsu: Stroke Therapy: Status of Anti-platelet Aggregation Drugs. Neurology 27:503, 1977.

28. D.J. Delessio - Editorial of Platelets, Their Antagonists, and Transient Cerebral Ischemia. JAMA 239:228, 1978.

29. J.C.M. Brust: Transient Ischemic Attacks: Natural History and Anticoagulation. Neurology 27:701, 1977.

30. M.A. Packham, J.P. Mustard: Clinical Pharmacology of Platelets. Blood 50:555-573, 1977.

31. H.J. Weiss, L.M. Aledorf: Impaired Platelets/Connective Tissue Reaction in Man After Aspirin Ingestion. Lancet, Volume II, pp. 495-497, 1967.

32. Harvey J. Weiss: Drug Therapy. New England Journal of Medicine, Part I, June 15, 1978, 1344-1347, Part II, June 22, 1978, 298:1403-1406.

33. Anturane Re-infarction Trail Research Group: Sulfinpyrazone in the Prevention of Cardiac Death After Myocardial Infarction: The Anturance Re-infarction Trial. New England Journal of Medicine 298:295, 1978.

34. P.R. Emmons, et al.: Effect of Dipyridamole on Human Platelet Behavior. Lancet, Volume II, pp. 603-606, 1965.

35. H.J. Weiss: Antiplatelet Drugs: A New Pharmacological Approach to the Prevention of Thrombosis. American Heart Journal 92:86-102, 1976.

36. W.S. Fields, N.A. Lemak, et al.: Controlled Trial of Aspirin in Cerebral Ischemia. Stroke 8:301, 1977.

37. A Randomized Trial of Aspirin and Sulfinpyrazone in Threatened Stroke. New England Journal of Medicine 299:53-59, 1978.

38. Francisco D. Cervantes, Lawrence J. Schneiderman, et al.: Anticoagulants In Cerebrovascular Disease: Critical Review of Studies. Archives of Internal Medicine 135: 875, June, 1975.

39. F.D. Cervantes and L.J. Schneiderman: Anticoagulants in Cerebrovascular Disease, A Critical Review of Studies. Archives of Internal Medicine 135:875, June, 1975.

40. J.E. Thompson: The Development of Carotid Artery Surgery. Archives of Surgery 107:643, 1973.

41. W.B. Chung, et al.: Long-term Results of Carotid Artery Surgery for Cerebrovascular Insufficiency. American Journal of Surgery 128:262, August, 1974.

42. J.E. Thompson, D.J. Austin, et al.: Carotid Endarterectomy for Cerebrovascular Insufficiency: Long-term results in 592 Patients Followed up to Thirteen Years. Annals of Surgery 172:663, October, 1970.

43. R.B. Bauer, J.S. Meyer, et al.: Joint Study of Extracranial Arterial Occlusion, III Progress Report of Controlled Study of Long-Term Survival in Patients with and without Operation. JAMA 208:509, 1969.

44. J.E. Thompson and C.M. Talkington: Surgical Progress in Carotid Endarterectomy. Annals of Surgery 184:1, July, 1976.

45. R.J. Hays, S.A. Levinson, et al.: Intraoperative Measurement of Carotid Back Pressure as a Guide to Operative Management for Carotid Endarterectomy. Surgery 72:953, December, 1972.

46. W.S. Fields - Editorial: Selection of Stroke Patients for Arterial Reconstructive Surgery. American Journal of Surgery 125:527, May, 1973.

47. J.E. Thompson, et al.: Management of Asymptomatic Carotid Bruits. The American Surgeon 42:77, February 1976.

48. C. Hachinski, et al.: Multi-Infarct Dementia: A Cause of Mental Deterioration in the Elderly. Lancet, 2:207, 1974.

49. D.K. Ziegler, R. Stephenson, et al.: Prognosis in Patients with Transient Ischemic Attacks. Stroke 4:666, 1973.

50. W.E. Stehbens: Pathology of the Cerebral Blood Vessels, C.V. Mosby, St. Louis, 1972.

51. R. Fogelholm, E. Kovalo, et al.: Transient G-A Syndrome, Analysis of 35 Cases. European Neurology, Volume 13, pp. 72-84, 1975.

52. R. Magaard and S. Ekestrom: The Influence of Arm Ischemia and Arm Hyperanemia on Subclavian and Vertebral Artery Blood Flow in Patients with Occlusive Disease of the Subclavian and Brachiocephalic Trunk. Scandinavian Journal of Thoracic Cardiovascular Surgery 9:240, 1975.

53. A. Humphries, J.R. Young, et al.: Relief of Vertebrobasilar Symptoms by Carotid Endarterectomy. Surgery 48:48, January, 1975.

54. J. McNamara, A. Heyman, et al.: The Value of Carotid Endarterectomy in Treating Transient Cerebral Ischemia of the Posterior Circulation. Neurology 27:682, 1977.

55. Cerebral Vasodilators Editorial. British Medical Journal 2:702, 1971.

CHAPTER II:

COMPLETED STROKE

GENERAL INFORMATION

A cerebral infarction is the sudden onset of a neurologic deficit caused by reduced or absent blood flow in the cerebral vessel. This vessel may be any one of the major vessels or any of their branches in the carotid or vertebral basilar system. Our diagnostic studies must confirm the absence of cerebral hemorrhage, neoplasm, or other space-occupying lesion which can be confused with cerebral infarction. While these symptoms develop rapidly over minutes, the progression of their severity can continue for a few hours without necessarily changing the diagnosis to that of thrombosis in evolution. The following case will illustrate that a completed stroke can have progression of the neurologic deficit.

A 65-year-old man developed some weakness in his right leg while walking to the kitchen sink to prepare for breakfast. He had been entirely asymptomatic until that time and had a history of moderate hypertension for which he was being treated. He returned to the kitchen table with some difficulty and sat down to make a phone call; he noticed difficulty dialing the telephone. He also had paresthesias in his right arm and leg.

He was taken to the hospital where, one hour later, he was found to have a moderate right hemiparesis with a mild right central facial weakness. There was decreased proprioception in the fingers of the right hand and in the toes of the right foot. There was also an extensor plantar response on the right side. During the course of the next 48 hours, there was little or no change in the patient's neurologic deficit; he had a completed stroke.

Cerebral infarction suggests a pathological structural abnormality which is irreversible. While this is so, the patient may recover his neurologic function entirely. This is because some of the damaged cells recover and resume their function. The collateral circulation is important in helping to improve the percentage of cells which are able to survive. For instance, the prognosis is generally better in a patient with internal carotid artery occlusion than in one with a middle cerebral artery occlusion. This is because the possibility for collateral circulation is better when the occlusion is in the internal carotid artery. Generally, the collateral circulation is better the further the occlusion is from the site of infarction. Clinically, we sometimes have difficulty localizing the exact site of pathology. Because of this, it is cogent to speak of infarction in the internal carotid or vertebral basilar artery distribution, rather than being more specific. In addition, it is imperative for therapeutic purposes that we differentiate between extra- and intracranial disease. Some vessels can definitely be identified as the site of pathology by virtue of the clinical picture. There are, of course, exceptions to the following examples.

LOCALIZABLE TYPES OF INFARCTION

When the internal carotid artery is thrombosed, there may be a hemiparesis which is contralateral to a Horner's syndrome (ptosis and miosis). The latter is secondary to sympathetic nerve involvement of the nerve fibers which wrap around the internal carotid artery and receive their blood supply from it. Loss of facial sweating does not occur because these sympathetic fibers are not involved.

The deficit caused by occlusion of the internal carotid artery, at times, is identical to that seen in occlusion of the middle cerebral artery. If a Horner's syndrome is present, this may be the only differentiating point. The presence of transient blindness, followed by a contralateral hemiparesis is an alternative syndrome which can be produced by internal carotid artery occlusion.

Occlusion of the anterior cerebral artery will produce primary weakness in the opposite lower extremity. Middle cerebral artery occlusion produces more weakness in the arm than in the leg.[1, 2, 3] (See Figures 2.1 and 2.2 for depiction of internal carotid system.)

The basilar artery is formed by the junction of the two vertebral arteries. They may supply equal amounts of blood to the basilar artery, but more often, the left vertebral artery supplies most of the blood. Occlusion of the nondominant vessel may be entirely asymptomatic. If the basilar artery is deprived of a critical amount of blood, any of the following lower brain stem syndromes, or combinations of them, may result. The lateral medullary infarction (Wallenberg's Syndrome) is probably the most common of these.

Infarction of the vertebral basilar system results from occlusion of:

1) the trunk of the vertebral or basilar artery
2) long circumferential vessels which are the posterior-inferior cerebellar artery, anterior-inferior cerebellar artery, or superior cerebellar artery
3) the paramedian vessels which supply a small wedge of brain stem on either side of the midline
4) short circumferential vessels which contribute to the supply of the lateral brain stem

There is overlap between these vessels and much variation from one person to the next.

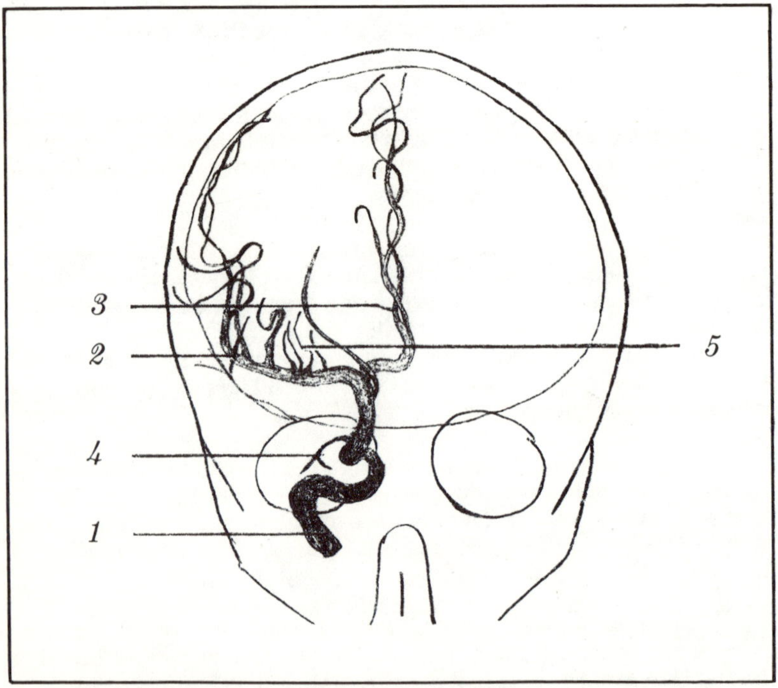

FIG. 2.1: Anterior view of internal carotid system: (1) Internal carotid artery; (2) Middle cerebral artery; (3) Anterior cerebral artery; (4) Ophthalmic artery; (5) Lenticulostriate artery.

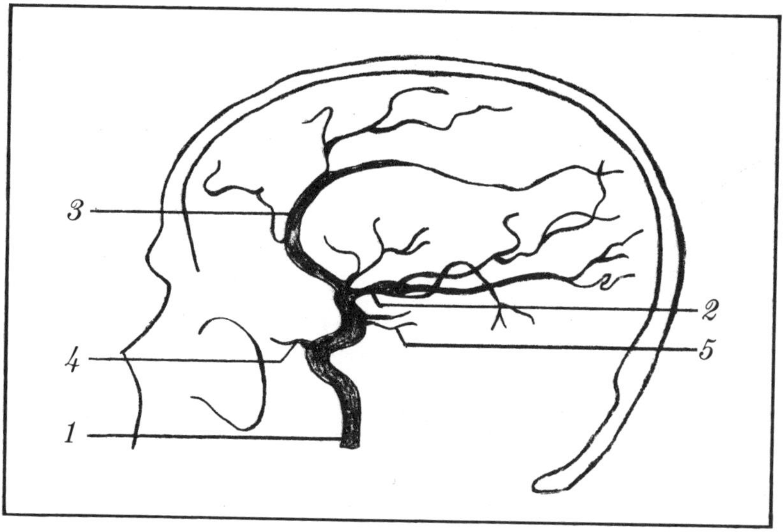

FIG. 2.2: Lateral view of internal carotid system: (1) Internal carotid artery; (2) Middle cerebral artery; (3) Anterior cerebral artery; (4) Opthalmic artery; (5) Posterior communicating artery.

The lateral medullary infarction has a characteristic neurologic picture. It may be caused by thrombosis in the posterior-inferior cerebellar artery or the vertebral artery (See Figure 2.3). These are the signs and symptoms:

1) cerebellar ataxia in the ipsilateral arm and leg

2) ipsilateral absent corneal reflex and/or decreased pain in the ipsilateral face in the first division of the trigeminal nerve

3) ipsilateral Horner's syndrome

4) dysphagia from infarction of the ipsilateral nucleus ambiguus

5) nystagmus from infarction of the vestibular nucleus

6) decreased pain and temperature in the contralateral arm and leg

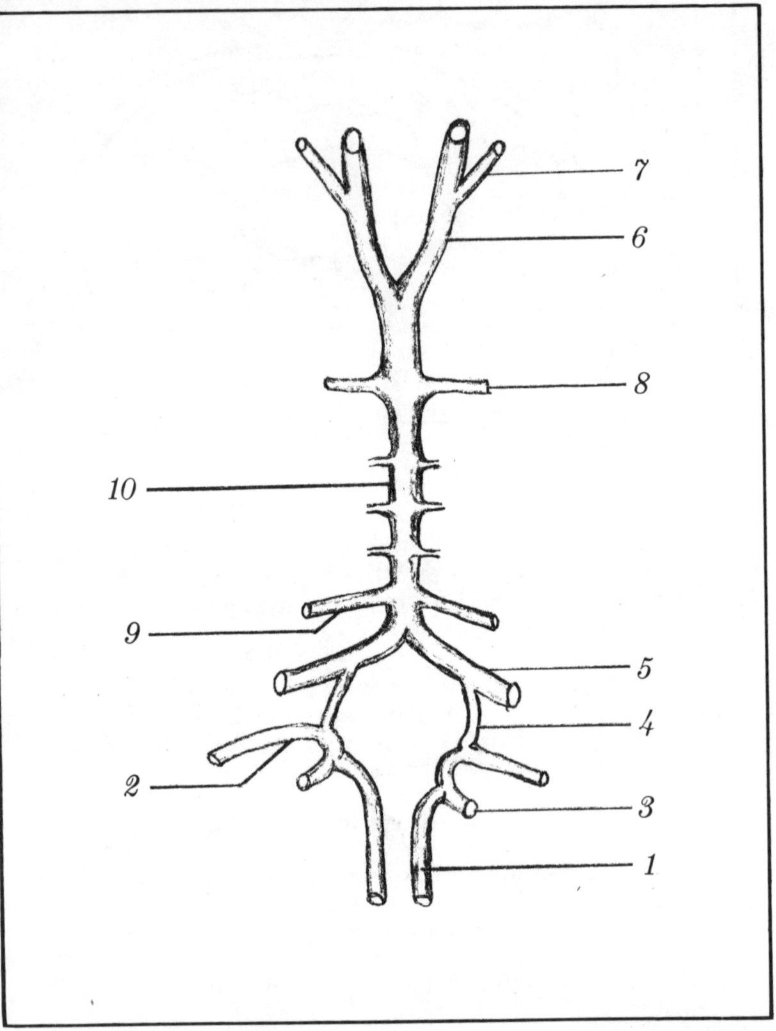

FIG. 2.3: Circle of Willis: (1) Internal carotid artery; (2) Middle cerebral artery; (3) Anterior cerebral artery; (4) Posterior communicating artery; (5) Posterior cerebral artery; (6) Vertebral artery; (7) Posterior inferior cerebellar artery; (8) Anterior inferior cerebellar artery; (9) Superior cerebellar artery; (10) Basilar artery.

The crossed syndrome, i.e., decreased sensation on one side of the face and the opposite extremities mentioned above is diagnostic of brain stem disease. In most instances the majority of these symptoms improve rather quickly after their onset. In rare cases, the dysphagia may persist to a severe degree requiring tracheotomy to prevent aspiration. In selected patients, section of the cricopharyngeal muscle may be helpful. This can be done if the dysphagia persists for several weeks and a cine-esophagram reveals a pharyngeal narrowing and delay in the passage of contrast media at the level of the cricopharyngeus muscle.

Thrombosis of the paramedian vessels produces a crossed syndrome characterized by paralysis of one of the cranial nerves with a midline nucleus, such as, the third, the sixth, or the twelfth and a contralateral hemiparesis.

The syndrome of infarction in the anterior-inferior cerebellar artery distribution consists of:

1) cerebellar ataxia in the ipsilateral arm and leg

2) impaired touch on the ipsilateral side of the face

3) ipsilateral Horner's syndrome (ptosis-miosis-anhydrosis)

4) ipsilateral peripheral seventh nerve weakness or paralysis

5) ipsilateral deafness

6) nystagmus

7) contralateral loss of pain and temperature in the extremities

The distinguishing features in this infarction is the loss of hearing and specifically, the dysfunction in the seventh and eighth cranial nerve as compared to the dysfunction in the tenth cranial nerve in the previously described syndrome of the posterior-inferior cerebellar artery infarction.

Infarction in the distribution of the superior cerebellar artery produces:

1) ipsilateral cerebellar ataxia with a dramatic intensity to the tremor

2) contralateral loss of pain and temperature in the face, arm, and leg

3) ipsilateral Horner's syndrome

This syndrome is much less commonly seen than the first two which have been described here.

Infarction in the distribution of the posterior cerebral artery is characterized by the following:

1) a contralateral homonymous hemianopia

2) contralateral loss of pain, temperature, proprioception, and vibratory sensation

3) contralateral hemiparesis which is incomplete and transient

In this syndrome, sensory symptoms and signs predominate over motor symptoms and signs. It is not uncommon for patients with this type of infarction to develop a hyperpathia, which is a very uncomfortable sensation in the involved extremities when they are touched.

The locked-in syndrome represents an infarction of the ventral pons, producing upper motor neuron paralysis to the muscles of articulation and swallowing together with a quadriplegia. Since the patients cannot talk, they are thought to be comatose. The patients are not deaf and they can respond to questions if a system is established. For instance, they can blink their eyes once for "no" and twice for "yes". It is obvious that the prognosis in these patients is very poor.

In most instances, there is little difficulty in making the diagnosis of a completed stroke. On occasion, this may be confused with a small intracerebral hemorrhage. In the past, differentiation depended upon the presence or absence of blood in the cerebrospinal fluid. We are often fooled unless a small hemorrhage is in close proximity to the arachnoid surface thus allowing blood to find its way into the cerebrospinal fluid. The use of computerized tomography scanning has eliminated this problem. This differentiation is important because it is not necessary to search for an extracranial lesion in the presence of an intracerebral hemorrhage.

There are certain symptoms that allow us to definitely make a diagnosis involving either the carotid or vertebral basilar system. It is important to make this differentiation for therapeutic and prognostic reasons. Monocular blindness, aphasia, and cortical sensory abnormalities (astereognosis, extinction to pin, and position sense) are always related to carotid artery ischemia. Hemisensory deficit and hemiparesis are most frequently related to carotid artery ischemia but can rarely occur in vertebral basilar disease. Homonymous hemianopia can occur in either system. Bilateral blindness, vertigo, dysphagia, diplopia, quadriparesis, deafness, ataxia, and crossed syndromes are characteristic of vertebral basilar disease.

Dementia has been attributed to cerebrovascular disease. It is clear at this time that most patients with dementia have an enzymatic defect related to Alzheimer's disease rather than cerebral arteriosclerosis. When vascular disease causes dementia, it is because of damage to a large area or to multiple areas of the cerebral hemispheres.[4,5]

As mentioned previously, it is sometimes necessary to differentiate intracerebral hemorrhage from cerebral infarction. Headaches occur more frequently and are more severe in patients with intracerebral hemorrhage than in those with ischemic infarctions. The same can be said for hypertension. The classic intracerebral hemorrhage usually presents with a moderately severe headache and progressive contralateral neurologic deficit, i.e., hemiparesis, homonymous hemianopia, and hemisensory deficit. This is followed promptly by a significant decrease in the level of consciousness as well as the development of bilateral Babinski signs. This is the description of a relatively large intracerebral hematoma. The rapid progression should alert the physician to the correct diagnosis. In this situation, computerized tomography is diagnostic. Lumbar puncture can be dangerous because of transtentorial herniation, which frequently occurs in patients with large intracerebral hemorrhages.

If a sudden onset of neurologic deficit cannot be documented, the diagnosis of cerebral infarction should not be made. It must be assumed that the diagnosis is not infarction until it can be proven. Occasionally, subdural hematomas are diagnosed erroneously as cerebral infarctions, because only the rapidly progressive phase of the disease is recognized. If a complete history were available, it would be seen that in almost all patients with subacute subdural hematoma there is a gradual progression of signs and symptoms over several days. The early insidious progression is missed in those patients who are diagnosed as having cerebral infarction.

On rare occasions, the patients with tumors present with catastrophic onset, presumably from hemorrhage into the tumor, vascular compression by the tumor causing infarction, or tumor emboli. Computerized tomography scanning will often make the differentiation. The presence of cerebrospinal fluid protein in the range of 100 mg.% or higher should alert the physician to the possible presence of a brain tumor.

NATURAL HISTORY

In understanding the natural history of cerebrovascular disease, we must first realize that transient ischemic attack in the distribution of a specific artery often gives warning of an infarction in that distribution. In one series a cerebral infarction occurred in one-third of patients with transient ischemic attacks. Fifty percent of all infarctions occurred within the first year after the transient ischemic attack. Twenty-one percent occurred during the month after the first attack.[16, 17, 18] For that reason, it is important to diagnose transient ischemic attacks and to investigate them thoroughly. This correlation is much more striking in carotid artery ischemia than in vertebral basilar ischemia. There is a seven percent mortality within 48 hours of a cerebral infarction with a 25 to 35 percent mortality after fourteen days in most series of hospitalized patients.[19, 20, 22] In order to predict the immediate survival from an infarction, the patient's level of consciousness is very important. Patients who are in a comatose state for longer than several hours have a very poor prognosis. In supratentorial infarctions, the state of consciousness is proportional to the magnitude of the cerebral damage.

Long-term morbidity may be more susceptible to change from therapeutic modalities than short-term morbidity. This latter may be affected most strongly by preventative measures. There appears to be an average death rate of 15 percent per year in patients who have had cerebral infarctions.[21, 22] This mortality appears to be strongly related to hypertension and cardiac disease. Treatment of hypertension can prolong survival. The more significant the hypertension, the shorter the long-term survival. Twenty-five to fifty percent of patients with cerebral infarction will have repeat infarction. Heart disease, in the form of cardiac failure, coronary artery disease, arrhythmia or other electrocardiographic changes, worsens the prognosis. Death occurs from another infarction in only about one-quarter of the patients. The major causes of death are myocardial infarction and congestive heart failure.[22, 23, 24, 25]

PREDISPOSING FACTORS

As mentioned previously atherosclerosis is involved in, if not the cause of, most cerebral infarctions. The pathogenesis of atherosclerosis seems to be related to platelets and their interaction with endothelial cells, serum lipids and their deposition, and to smooth muscle cell proliferation in the arterial wall. These factors interact to produce the pathologic condition.[6, 7, 8, 9] The primary initiating event is not universally agreed upon. Some authors suggest that platelet adherence to the endothelium is the initiating event causing damage to the cell and enabling lipid to gain entrance into the vessel wall. These authors also feel that hyperlipidemia causes increased platelet adherence and increased lipid deposition.[10] Many authors, and perhaps the majority at this time, feel that smooth muscle cell proliferation and collagen production is of prime importance. This seems to be related to lipids in the form of low density lipoprotein and very low density lipoprotein entering the smooth muscle cells.[11] These cells seem to be selectively the sight of lipid deposition. They proliferate and migrate into the arterial intima. The lipid, as well as tissue factors, some of which seem to be elaborated by platelets, seem to be important in this cell proliferation. It can be seen that many factors are brought into play, and there is a complex interaction between platelets, endothelial cells, muscle cells, and lipid in the pathogenesis of atherosclerosis. Perhaps the muscle cell and lipid are the two most important factors.[12]

We do not know whether there is one factor which begins the pathologic process and is necessary for it. It is obvious that genetic factors are important as are dietary components. Factors such as hypertension and coagulation function have a role in accelerating the process partially, but not exclusively, by means of causing endothelial damage. It has also been shown that if serum lipid levels can be maintained at sustained low levels for prolonged periods of time the development of an atheroma can be inhibited, and those that have developed can also be seen to regress.[13, 14, 15, 42, 43]

It is recognized that there is increase in cerebral infarction with age. A genetic predisposition to vascular disease also exists. This most likely relates to the ease and age of formation of the atheroma in cerebral vessels.[30, 31] There are many other factors which seem to predispose a patient to cerebral infarction. Next to age and genetics, hypertension is definitely the most important of these.[26, 27, 28, 29, 32] It is this factor that is most frequently associated with increased frequency of infarction. This frequency appears to be proportional to the systolic and diastolic blood pressures. There probably have been too few patients studied with isolated systolic hypertension; however, there is a strong suggestion that it is as important as diastolic hypertension in the correlation with ischemic cerebrovascular disease.[33] At one time, it was felt that the correlation was much stronger in patients under fifty years of age. This did not seem to be the case, and the correlation persists regardless of age or sex of the patient. Hypertension appears to cause accelerated arterial intimal damage and in that way, and perhaps others, it accelerates atherosclerosis.[26] It may also decrease cerebral blood flow through other mechanisms such as cerebral arterial spasm. It has become clear that hypertension should be treated in almost all patients, even in those where the abnormality seems to be primarily in systolic blood pressure. If blood pressure is lowered slowly to normal limits, the overwhelming majority of patients benefit with decreased vascular morbidity.

Hypertension is strongly implicated in lacunar infarctions. These are small cavities seen in the brain at post-mortem examination. They are usually no more than $1\frac{1}{2}$ cm. in diameter and are most frequently only a few millimeters in diameter. They are most likely formed by the occlusion of a small intracranial arterial segment causing a micro-infarction.[34, 35, 40] Rarely, are they related to occlusion of a Charcot Bouchard microaneurysm. In rare instances, they may be caused by small localized hemorrhages from one of these microaneurysms. They are most frequently seen in the putamen and globus pallidus followed by the pons, thalmus, and caudate nucleus. They are also found frequently in the white matter. Clinically, the patient develops a sudden neurologic deficit which does not progress and which rapidly improves, though, not always completely. The literature contains several syndromes which have been seen in lacunar infarctions. As our experience becomes greater, it seems that the etiology of these syndromes are not necessarily confined to discrete lacunar infarctions. The syndromes include a pure hemisensory deficit due to a thalamic lacun.[37] Pure motor hemiplegia has also been reported.[36] Cerebellar signs and pyramidal signs in one arm and leg or in one extremity has also been reported.[38] Dysarthria and one clumsy hand is yet another syndrome present in the literature.[39] When there are multiple bilateral lacunar infarctions, a pseudobulbar palsy results. This is a weakness of the muscles innervated by the lower brain stem, such as the muscles of the tongues, lips, and pharynx. This produces dysphagia and dysarthria. The dysfunction is located in the corticobulbar tracts which connect with the lower motor neuron. The patients with pseudobulbar palsy also demonstrate uncontrollable laughing or crying produced by minimal emotional stimuli.

The association of blood lipids in cerebral infarction is considerably weaker. Both hypercholesterolemia and hypertriglyceridemia have been implicated in having a role in increased incidence of cerebral infarction. This seems to be more important in men and generally in patients under sixty years of age.[7, 41]

Cholesterol appears to have a higher correlation than does triglyceride. In the absence of other complicating factors, however, its correlation is not strong.[44] Recently it has been pointed out that low values of high density lipoprotein cholesterol may have a significant relationship to vascular disease and specifically to cerebrovascular disease. Although this has not been studied as carefully as in coronary artery disease, the correlation certainly appears to exist.[45] There are hypotheses on how high density lipoproteins may be protective to a patient. It has been suggested that low density lipoprotein is prevented from entering the intima of blood vessels by the presence of high density lipoprotein. It may also in some way stimulate lipolysis and may increase lipid transport from the cells.

Patients with impaired glucose tolerance also have a high risk of cerebral infarction. It is thought that this increased risk is in excess of that caused by the increased incidence of hypertension and hyperlipidemia in patients with diabetes.[27] The more severe the diabetes, the greater is the risk of cerebral infarction.

Various types of cardiac abnormalities also play a significant role. Coronary artery disease has a positive correlation as does congestive heart failure. Electrocardiographic abnormalities including arrhythmias and left ventricular abnormalities as well as an enlarged heart are also important. Cardiac disease is an important cause of death in patients after cerebral infarction, both early and late. It has been found that some patients with cerebral infarction have abnormal coagulation studies which may also predispose them to having thrombosis of an artery.[46, 47]

Less significant factors are obesity, which is important primarily due to its aggravation of hypertension and hyperlipidemia. Smoking may also be a factor, but it appears to be more important in men and in younger age groups. Oral contraceptives may increase the likelihood of a cerebral infarction in some young women, particularly in those who are heavy smokers or who have migraine headaches.[48, 49] Much of the problem seems to be caused by contraceptives with high estrogen content. There are a number of experts in the field who feel that even the newer contraceptives increase the risk of cerebral infarction in patients taking them.

Since the most effective management of cerebral infarction at this time seems to be its prevention, attention must be given to how we can alter its development. Hypertension should be controlled with medication as should diabetes.[50] While optimal diabetic control does not seemingly decrease other nervous system complications such as peripheral neuropathy, it does appear to be an important factor in counteracting the effect that diabetes has on increasing the frequency of cerebral infarction. Of course, therapeutic hypoglycemia is to be avoided because it may carry an even higher risk of cerebral damage in the elderly.

The lipids in the serum are both endogenous and exogenous. Nevertheless, reduction of cholesterol and triglyceride intake may be an important way of reducing the serum levels. Additional help can be gained from medication such as clofibrate and cholestyramine where these drugs are indicated. Other drugs have been used experimentally including pyridinol carbamate.[14, 15, 42, 43] There is evidence that existing atheromata can decrease in size with proper pharmacologic and dietary therapy.

DIAGNOSTIC STUDIES

As part of the evaluation of the patient who has had an acute cerebral infarction, the following studies should be done. Of course, the patient should have a thorough history and physical examination. A blood count should be performed looking for an elevated hematocrit or leukocytosis which could be signaling the presence of an infection. The former could predispose a patient to arterial or venous thrombosis. A fasting blood sugar and other tests of carbohydrate tolerance should be done in order to make a diagnosis of diabetes. An EKG should be performed looking for evidence of arrhythmia and left ventricular hypertrophy as well as other abnormalities. Serum lipids and a biochemical profile to include urea and electrolytes are also important. A chest x-ray to assess the cardiac size and pulmonary appearance must also be done. After an acute infarction, it is necessary to search for evidence that might suggest a hypoxic state either chronically or acutely. We must also be alert to the fact that acute pneumonia can cause hypoxia and confusion even without hypoxia in elderly patients complicating their management.

The following studies are also important in the evaluation of a patient with an acute cerebral infarction. Skull x-ray is often normal, but it is easily performed and may be diagnostic. There is little risk to the patient in doing this procedure. It will rapidly reveal evidence of significant pineal gland shift and show other conditions which might be confused with a cerebral infarction. The skull x-ray can show areas of abnormal tumor calcification or demineralization of the dorsum sellae suggesting chronically increased intracranial pressure. In most patients with cerebral infarction, the skull x-ray is normal unless the pineal gland is slightly shifted because of associated cerebral edema.

The electroencephalogram can confirm the location of infarction and can assess the functional integrity of the cerebral hemisphere. On occasion, the electroencephalographic abnormality may persist after the patient's neurologic examination has returned to normal. EEG has little value in evaluating patients with infarctions involving the vertebral basilar system. With the more frequent use of the evoked potential studies, we may find that more information is obtained and that this then has greater prognostic implication.

There are several other non-invasive studies which help us assess the cerebral circulation. These have been discussed in the chapter concerning transient ischemic attacks. Newer methods of cerebral blood flow determination are also being developed. The factor which seems to be most difficult and most important is the determination of regional rather than total cerebral blood flow. A good assessment of this value is very difficult to obtain and at the present time is not generally available.

Many patients with cerebral infarction require lumbar puncture. This is done in order to make our diagnostic considerations more precise. We perform the lumbar puncture in the lateral recumbent position to determine the pressure and the presence of red and white blood cells, proteins, and serology. If infection is suspected, of course, glucose would also be determined. Most patients with ischemic cerebral infarctions have normal spinal fluid examinations. Rarely, there may be a mildly elevated pressure and protein. In some instances, there may be a slight but probably insignificant lymphocytosis of less than ten cells per cubic millimeter. Occasionally, the finding of white blood cells and a positive serology would suggest the presence of meningovascular lues. This disease can also present as a cerebral infarction. Cerebrospinal fluid pleocytosis will also be seen in all types of meningitis. While significant protein elevation rarely can be seen in cerebral infarction, the finding of an elevation to 100 mg.% or more should at least lead to other diagnostic considerations.

Lumbar puncture should always be done in the lateral recumbent position preferably with a 20-gauge short bevel needle. We should worry about the potential for herniation when there is a major neurologic deficit and when the patient has a significant depression in his level of consciousness. When available, the computerized tomography scan is a must in this situation. A large ventricular shift with or without evidence of an infarction is a contraindication to a lumbar puncture.

The presence of transtentorial herniation is, of course, a contraindication to lumbar puncture, since the situation is life threatening and a lumbar puncture might aggravate it. We must remember that intracerebral hemorrhage and even cerebral infarctions can act as a mass lesion under the proper circumstances.

Uncal herniation is produced when the medial portion of the temporal lobe moves toward the midline and over the free edge of the tentorium. The first sign is the unilateral dilated pupil with a sluggish response to light and a decrease in the state of awareness. When the pupil becomes dilated and fixed, the remainder of the third nerve dysfunction develops quickly; then the patient has a more significant decrease in his level of consciousness. With progression, the patient develops bilateral brain stem dysfunction including bilateral pupillary changes, absent Doll's eye movement and respiratory abnormality, as well as decerebrate rigidity. Since the situation occurs as a slow continuum, it can be observed anywhere during its development. More commonly, patients with supratentorial masses have a central, rather than a lateral (uncal) herniation. Here the initial symptoms and signs seem to relate to diencephalic compression. The first sign is change in the patient's alertness. This usually leads to a progressive obtundation. There are frequent yawns, and periodic Cheyne-Stokes respirations develop. The pupils are initially small (1 to 3 mm.), equal and reactive to light with a small excursion of movement. If there was an original hemiparesis present due to a stroke, it may worsen. Tone increases bilaterally, and the patient may develop bilateral extensor plantar responses. Decorticate rigidity may also develop, and this may proceed to decerebrate rigidity which seems frequently to occur first on the side of the initial hemiplegia. The pupils may then become fixed in midposition, and the patient's condition deteriorates, eventually leading to respiratory arrest and death.

In the previous discussion, we mentioned both decorticate and decerebrate rigidity. In decorticate rigidity the patient has flexion of his arms, wrists, and fingers with adduction of the upper extremities and extension, internal rotation, and plantar flexion in the lower extremities. With fully developed decerebrate rigidity, the upper extremities are stiffly extended, adducted and are hyperpronated. The legs are stiffly extended, and the feet are plantar flexed. Often it is necessary to administer a noxious stimulus in order to produce the complete picture of decerebrate rigidity.

Dynamic radio isotope studies have rarely been helpful, in some patients with cerebral infarction, in showing a major vessel occlusion. The static brain scan is most often normal for at least 48 to 72 hours after the infarction. After this period of time, it frequently becomes abnormal giving some idea of the size of the infarction. It does not, however, distinguish between cerebral infarction and hemorrhage and does not show the presence of cerebral edema associated with an infarction. For this reason, CT scanning is much more valuable because it allows us to easily assess these factors. It shows us the brain anatomy and evidence of lateral and perhaps downward herniation. It must be remembered that with the computerized tomography scan, it may also take as long as 72 hours for an abnormality associated with cerebral infarction to become easily identifiable. It is desirable to perform computerized tomography scanning of the brain without the use of intravenous iodinated contrast media. When this is done, its safety is the same as that of a skull x-ray. When contrast media is injected, we then add the risk of a reaction to the iodinated media. This is admittedly a small risk, but nevertheless, a definite one.[51] There is also a small group of patients in whom the cerebral infarction can be better identified following the injection of contrast media. An even smaller group of patients exists in whom the infarction is obscured by the injection of contrast media, because the media makes the infarction appear to be isodense with the surrounding normal brain substance. This procedure is not as effective in evaluating brain stem infarction.

At one time, it was thought that a significant increase in radiodensity of an abnormality following an injection of contrast media was characteristic of neoplasms. It is evident that cerebral infarction can demonstrate this characteristic as well. It may also show evidence of a mass effect; and in these instances, the differentiation between neoplasm and infarction may rest strongly on the patient's history or on the performance of serial CT scans. With serial scans, infarction will improve; and there may be enlargement of a neoplasm. At this time, there is no doubt that computerized axial tomography of the brain is the most effective non-invasive procedure available to use for the diagnosis of supratentorial and infratentorial abnormalities.

UNUSUAL CAUSES OF STROKE

While the overwhelming majority of cerebral infarctions are related to atherosclerosis, there are less common etiologies. Anatomical variation in the carotid artery such as looping and kinking has been implicated. Most physicians, including this author, feel that these are asymptomatic and are not the cause of central nervous system symptoms. Another condition which has recently been recognized with increased frequency, is fibromuscular hyperplasia. It is a process of unknown etiology which involves elements of the intima and media of large arteries. It was first recognized in the renal artery but has been found, on several occasions, to involve the carotid artery and less commonly some of its intracranial branches. It is a localized "beading" of the vessel with very short areas of constriction alternating with dilatation of equally short length. This process often causes stenosis of the vessel lumen and most frequently involves only short segments at a time. The process is more common in women, and the natural history is not well known. The process, however, does cause strokes in relatively young patients. Definitive diagnosis can be made by angiography.[52] Multiple narrowing in major branches of the aorta develop from different etiologies. Many of the early cases were associated with the loss of arterial pulsations in the head, neck, and arms and were often associated with bruits. Many of the first reports of this problem were in young Oriental women. They had an arteritis which was sometimes associated with giant cells. Syphilitic aortitis, with or without aneurysm formation, was another cause. Moyamoya disease is a rare condition which occurs most frequently in young female patients. It consists of attenuation of both carotid arteries and its branches in the circle of Willis. There is also the development of a fine network of anastomotic channels from which the cerebrum receives most of its blood supply. The etiology of this problem is unknown and there are proponents of both the developmental and acquired etiology for it.[53, 55]

Trauma to the carotid artery or sudden violent stretching causing an intimal tear has been reported to cause complete thrombosis of the vessel. Inflammation can spread from the retropharyngeal area and can cause carotid artery occlusion as can vasculitis secondary to infections such as tuberculosis, syphilis, and mucor mycosis.[54] When there is cerebrovascular occlusion in collagen vascular disease, it is much more likely to be related to lupus erythematosus than to polyarteritis.[56]

Polycythemia has been reported to cause ischemic cerebrovascular disease in patients with elevated hematocrits regardless of whether the process is primary or secondary. With increases in hematocrit over 55 percent, there begins to be a significant increase in blood viscosity as well as in peripheral resistance. In secondary forms, there may also be hypoxemia to complicate the picture. In polycythemia vera, abnormal platelet function may contribute to the propensity for ischemic vascular symptomatology.[56]

Recurrent cerebral infarction may occur in up to 25 percent of patients with sickle cell anemia. Other hemoglobinopathies may cause this problem to a much lesser degree. Of course, other diseases of blood elements and serum proteins which cause a hypercoagulable or hyperviscous state predispose to cerebral infarction. Patients with homocystinuria, which is an unusual inborn error of metabolism, have an inordinate number of arterial thromboses. These patients have a Marfan-like habitus with long extremities and fingers, as well as dislocated ocular lenses.

There are patients who develop cerebral infarction during an attack of cerebrovascular spasm with migraine headaches; fortunately, this is rare. There is also an unusual group of patients who develop cerebral infarction in the last month of pregnancy or shortly after delivery. The etiology of this situation is not always clear, and it does not always seem to be related to a hypercoagulable state. At one time, it was hypothesized that the problem was in the venous system; however, in most instances it appears to be related to arterial occlusion.

TREATMENT OF ACUTE INFARCTION

The therapy of acute cerebral infarction is initially in the realm of preventative medicine, in that we treat factors which seem to predispose patients to cerebral infarction. It is also our goal to limit the extent of the infarction, if possible, once it has developed. In other words, we wish to decrease the ultimate morbidity and shorten the period during which the patient's neurologic deficit is most severe. The security of a patient's airway is of prime importance, and it must be protected even if this means endotracheal intubation or tracheotomy. It is necessary to provide adequate oxygenation, insure against aspiration, and clear the airway of secretions. In mild cerebral infarctions, this is not a problem, but in patients with obtundation and dysphagia, it requires special attention. If the patient has difficulty swallowing, he should be given nothing by mouth that could present an opportunity for aspiration and its consequences. Atelectasis can also be a problem, particularly in a partially paralyzed patient with or without a decreased level of consciousness; this can ultimately lead to bronchopneumonia. Some authorities feel that inhalation of 30 to 40% oxygen helps to decrease cerebral anoxia. Prolonged use of 100% oxygen is to be discouraged because of its toxic effects on the bronchial tree and also because it produces cerebral vasoconstriction.[57] Hyperbaric oxygen has been used, but there does not appear to be any sustained benefit from it; and it is an expensive form of therapy which is not generally available.

There are autoregulatory mechanisms which maintain cerebral blood flow at adequate levels despite changes, particularly drops in systemic blood pressure. The vascular tone of the cerebral vessels responds to changes in pressure as well as to changes in carbon dioxide and pH. When a patient has had an acute cerebral vascular accident, autoregulation in the infarcted area is lost, and the patient's cerebral blood flow appears to be directly proportional to his systemic blood pressure. There also appears to be a loss of responsiveness to chemical agents such as carbon dioxide, which is known to be a potent dilator of normally reacting cerebral blood vessels. At one time, there was widespread interest in the use of 3 to 5% carbon dioxide inhalation in order to dilate cerebral blood vessels in the region of an acute cerebral infarction. It then became apparent that the vasculature in the region of the infarction is maximally dilated shortly after the onset of symptoms. The involved vasculature is not responsive to the carbon dioxide. Uninvolved vessels in areas around the infarction will be more responsive to the carbon dioxide and will, therefore, dilate. The blood will flow from areas of higher pressure to areas of lower pressure. Prior to the institution of carbon dioxide, maximal flow was going into the area of the infarction where the vessels were dilated. When the normal blood vessels also became dilated secondary to the carbon dioxide, the pressure and resistance differential was lost; and there is reason to believe that blood flow within the infarcted area could be decreased. This process is referred to as a "steal". Theoretically, blood flows into normal areas at the expense of the infarcted areas.[58] While this appears to be a rational explanation, it has not been conclusively shown. CO_2 has not benefited patients in any way and should not be used.

Hyperventilation with reduction of $PaCO_2$ has been used, since it was thought that decreased level of carbon dioxide would cause a situation in which blood could be diverted from normal brain to the infarcted area. It was thought that the mechanism would be just the opposite of that previously described, with constriction rather than dilation of the normal blood vessels. The procedure has not been shown to be effective in decreasing the morbidity in a patient with acute cerebral infarction.[59]

Drugs have been used for cerebral vasodilation in acute infarctions. Most vasodilators effectively dilate peripheral vessels; but in doing so, they may cause a drop in blood pressure with a concomitant decreased cerebral blood flow. Papaverine has been shown to increase cerebral blood flow when given intravenously. Some investigators have found improvement in neurologic deficit. Others, however, have shown increased cerebral blood flow without documenting improvement in their patients. The danger of dilating normal vessels and decreasing the pressure flow differential is the same with Papaverine as it is with carbon dioxide. We do not recommend the use of vasodilators at this time.[60]

Low molecular weight Dextran may be of value in protecting the patient's cerebral circulation by decreasing blood viscosity and platelet adhesiveness. There may be a nonspecific effect related to expanding the blood volume. Evidence of significant improvement is scanty.[61]

Cerebral edema may be a major cause of death in patients with acute infarctions by producing cerebral herniation. Corticosteroids have been recommended for management of this problem; there is sentiment both for and against their effectiveness. It is generally agreed that this drug is not as effective in treating edema associated with cerebral infarction as it is in treating the edema associated with a cerebral neoplasm. Likewise, it has not been effective in significantly decreasing the neurologic deficit associated with this pathology. Dexamethasone has been used in a dose of 10 mg. initially followed by 4 mg. every six hours. Some attention is being given to other larger doses; it may be more effective, but these studies are still in a very early stage. The steroids should be continued for a period of four to five days.[62, 63]

Glycerol has also been used for the purpose of decreasing cerebral edema; its value is controversial. It has been used in a dose of one gram per kilogram, orally four times daily. When given intravenously in a 10% solution, it has been reported, on occasion, to cause hemolysis. It appears to act, at least partially, because of its properties as an osmotic diuretic.[64, 65]

Attention should be paid to the patient's blood pressure acutely. If the patient has evidence of hypotension, this is <u>not</u> related to the intracranial pathology; the source of the hypotension must be found. It is often secondary to intra-abdominal bleeding or a myocardial infarction. Attempts must be made to restore the blood pressure to normal, in these patients, in order to maintain an adequate cerebral blood flow.

The blood pressure is often transiently elevated with acute intracranial infarction in previously normotensive patients. This appears to be a homeostatic mechanism in order to improve blood flow; <u>no therapy</u> for the increased blood pressure is indicated acutely in these patients. An even more common problem is faced when a patient with known hypertension develops cerebral infarction. In this situation there is often a dramatic rise in both systolic and diastolic pressures. If the patient was previously receiving medication, it should be continued at the same dosage. If the patient was not previously receiving therapy, <u>none</u> should be given for 48 to 72 hours. Any sudden drop in blood pressure from medication can increase the damage to the infarcted area. After 48 to 72 hours, medication can be used to slowly lower the blood pressure. Increased intracranial pressure is seen both with cerebral hemorrhages and with infarctions. In these patients, the increased blood pressure is necessary to maintain cerebral blood flow; and there should be a greater delay in the institution of antihypertensive medications.[50, 66]

The patient should receive adequate hydration and no effort should be made to dehydrate the patient by withholding fluids. Serum electrolytes and osmolality should be watched because inappropriate ADH secretion can develop. If this goes unrecognized and significant hyponatremia develops, a decrease in the patient's level of consciousness or a convulsive seizure may develop.

Seizures develop in seven percent of patients with thrombotic infarction and should be treated promptly.[67] This occurs even with no electrolyte disturbance. Because of the risk of seizures, some physicians advocate prophylactic anticonvulsant medication in patients with large infarctions, particularly when cerebral cortical involvement is suspected. The drug of choice in these patients is Dilantin, because it does not decrease their level of consciousness. Seizures, developing several months after a cerebral infarction, are not an uncommon situation particularly with cortical infarctions. These patients are seen in the emergency room with a recrudescence or worsening of their previous neurologic deficit. This actually represents a Todd's paralysis following a seizure, and the deficit should be returned to the premorbid level in 24 to 48 hours.

Angiography is to be discouraged in patients with acute cerebral infarction, unless it is necessary to distinguish infarction from other diagnostic considerations. This has become even less necessary since the use of computerized tomography scanning. There is a definite risk in worsening the patient's deficit when angiography is performed in the presence of an acute cerebral infarction. After the acute period has passed, angiography is indicated if the patient has a reasonable or complete recovery from his deficit. This applies only to carotid system strokes. The necessity for this approach is to establish the presence of a surgically correctable lesion in the involved carotid artery extracranially. The subsequent removal of this lesion, i.e., ulcerated plaque or stenotic lesion with ulceration will prevent recurrent strokes in some patients.

There is no convincing evidence that long-term anticoagulation with Coumadin or heparin is of any value to patients with completed strokes. Since this is so, it is not worth the risk of anticoagulation to use these medications. Recently, however, there has been a suggestion that the use of aspirin in the dose of five grains q.i.d. might decrease the frequency of recurrent strokes in men. It is not clear why this therapy was not effective in women; it appears that further investigation is necessary in this area.[68]

Neurosurgery is rarely indicated in cerebral infarction. Patients with a large cerebellar infarction are an exception because the cerebellum may swell causing significant pressure on the brain stem. Unless the swollen infarcted cerebellum is removed, the patient may die from brain stem compression. Computerized tomography scanning greatly increases our accuracy in establishing the diagnosis of a cerebellar infarction.

It can be seen that our efforts to date have fallen into a pattern of trial and error. We do not have an agreed upon method of treatment for patients with significant cerebral infarction that will clearly decrease morbidity and improve chances of recovery. Such a therapy certainly is to be desired; however, further experimental work will be necessary before we can definitely perform a major role in altering the outcome of ischemic infarction.

CASE STUDIES

CASE 1:

A 62-year-old white male was seen in a local doctor's office for evaluation. The local physician noted the patient had bilateral carotid bruits and was going to admit him to the hospital for evaluation of the problem. The following day the family called the physician to tell him that the patient was having some difficulty with his speech. One hour later he was referred to the hospital emergency room, and was seen approximately at 1:30 p. m. At that time, neurological examinations revealed the patient to have a global aphasia. There was no definite motor weakness present. Extraocular muscle movements were normal. The patient was alert. The optic discs were flat. There was a short soft systolic bruit over the right carotid artery at the angle of the jaw. There were no bruits heard over the left carotid artery despite the fact that the family physician was aware that a bruit had been present previously. There was a thrill and a long loud systolic bruit over the left subclavian artery. There was no carotid pulse felt in the left neck. The left superficial temporal artery was not palpable. Blood pressure was 140/90 in the left arm and 80/60 in the right arm. There was a pulse delay at the right radial pulse compared to the left.

At the time of our evaluation we felt the patient had a total occlusion of his left common carotid artery. A lumbar puncture was immediately done; the fluid was crystal clear without any microscopic red blood cells. Coagulation studies were normal. Intravenous heparin was started immediately via the bolus technique. Electrocardiogram was normal. Chest x-ray was normal. Within one hour of starting the heparin, the patient's speech improved except for a definite moderate anomic aphasia. He still had no other focal neurological symptoms or signs. Blood studies revealed an increase in triglycerides and cholesterol with no other abnormalities being noted, except for a blood sugar of 220 mg.%. The patient was known to have an adult onset of diabetes but followed only a diet for this problem. The following day the patient's aphasia persisted without change, and a computerized tomography scan done at that time was within normal limits. After five days of heparin therapy, the patient's neurological status had remained stable. We elected to proceed with an aortic arch study. The heparin was stopped and an aortic arch study was done. The latter was supplemented by individual studies of both common carotid arteries and internal carotid arteries in the neck and intracranially. This study revealed total occlusion of the left common carotid artery. Despite the thrill and the bruits, no significant lesion was seen over the left subclavian artery. The innominate artery was normal. There was total occlusion of the right subclavian artery. Selective study of the right common carotid artery revealed an ulcerating plaque at the origin and on the posterior wall of the right internal carotid artery. As the dye progressed intracranially, it was noted that the posterior cerebral artery was a branch off the internal carotid artery. The dye went from the carotid artery to the posterior cerebral artery, and retrograde down the right vertebral artery to supply blood to the right arm in an attempt to compensate for the total thrombosis of the right subclavian artery. We felt that this vertebral steal was diverting some blood from the patient's carotid circulation, and that the right carotid circulation was absolutely necessary to give us good collateral circulation to the left brain. The right carotid circulation intracranially revealed good collateral filling on the left side through the circle of Willis.

It was elected to carry out an axillary-axillary bypass in order to equalize the blood pressure in both arms. It was hoped that this improvement in the circulation of the right arm would decrease the vertebral steal noted in the carotid study and allow for better collateral circulation in the brain. The procedure was carried out without any adverse effects. The patient was discharged on aspirin, 650 mg. twice a day. At the time of discharge he continued to have a mild anomic aphasia but no other focal neurological deficit was present. There is no other focal neurological deficit was present. There is no long-term follow up available on this patient at this time, but one month after surgery his blood pressure was 135/90 in both arms.

::

CASE 2:

A 68-year-old white male was seen in the emergency room because of a sudden unsteady gait that occurred on arising that morning. Neurological examination revealed the patient to have a wide-based gait, with falling to the left. There were no other neurological abnormalities noted at the time of admission. There were no appendicular cerebellar signs. There were no cranial nerve abnormalities or sensory changes. His blood pressure was 150/90 in the left arm and 155/95 in the right arm. There were no neck bruits present. The patient was known to be a diabetic for fourteen years and took one Diabinese tablet daily and followed a diet. Blood sugar in the emergency room was 220 mg.%. Skull x-ray was normal.

SMA-12 was normal except for a cholesterol of 350 mg.%. The electrocardiogram was normal. There were no heart murmurs present. He was admitted to the hospital and seen five hours later by the resident. At that time, it was noted that he had a left Horner's syndrome and an absent left corneal reflex. There were moderate appendicular cerebellar signs in the left arm and left leg. There was paralysis of the left side of the uvula on phonation. He had significant dysphagia and hoarseness. There was hyperesthesia to pin involving the right arm, the right side of the body and the right leg.

It was clear that the patient's cerebellar deficit, noted at the time of admission to the emergency room, had proceeded to a full blown Wallenberg's syndrome when seen five hours later in the hospital. Since the clinical picture represented a thrombosis, either of the left vertebral artery, left posterior-inferior cerebellar artery, heparin therapy was not started. The following morning it was apparent that he was having a great deal of difficulty handling his secretions, and he was unable to swallow either liquids or semi-solid food. Computerized tomography scan at that time was normal. Spinal fluid examination was normal. The same day, a tracheotomy was done and was cuffed to prevent aspiration. At this time, his blood pressure dropped to 130/80 in both arms without any specific therapy.

His course in the hospital was characterized by improvement in the cerebellar deficit in the left arm and leg. He was able to ambulate quite well with a walker. His dysphagia persisted to a significant degree and the sensory changes were as recorded previously.

Subsequently, a cine-esophogram was done that revealed spasm of the cricopharyngeus muscle. Under local anesthesia, the cricopharyngeus muscle was sectioned; within the next several days, the patient's swallowing improved, and within a week, the swallowing returned to normal. The tracheostomy tube was subsequently removed. At the time of discharge, a residual left Horner's syndrome and decreased sensation to pin and temperature in the right arm, body and leg were present. The other neurological symptoms had disappeared except for a weakness of the left side of the palate. He was discharged on aspirin, 650 mg. twice a day.

This case illustrates how a completed stroke may take several hours to evolve completely. Had the patient shown any progression from the time his Wallenberg's syndrome had reached its maximum, intravenous therapy with heparin would have been started immediately.

::

REFERENCES

1. C.M. Fisher: Occlusion of the Internal Carotid Artery. AMA, Archives of Neurology and Psychiatry 65:346-77, 1951.

2. F. McDowell, J. Potes, S. Groch: The Natural History of Internal Carotid and Vertebral-Basilar Artery Occlusion. Neurology 11:153-7, 1961.

3. C.M. Fisher, I. Gore, N. Okabe, D.D. White: Atherosclerosis of the Carotid and Vertebral Arteries - Extracranial and Intracranial. Journal of Neuropathology and Experimental Neurology 24:55-76, 1965.

4. V.C. Hachinsky, N.A. Lessen, J. Marshal: Multi-Infarct Dementia. Lancet, Volume II, pp. 207-10, 1974.

5. C.D. Marsden, M.J.G. Harrison: Outcome of Investigation of Patients with Presenile Dementia. British Medical Journal 1:249, 1972.

6. H.F. Hoff, C.C. Heiderman, R.L. Jackson: Localization Patterns of Plasma Apolipoproteins in Human Atherosclerotic Lesions. Circulation Research 37:72-9, 1975.

7. G.S. Getz, D. Vesselinovitch, R.W. Wissler: A Dynamic Pathology of Atherosclerosis. American Journal of Medicine, 46:185, 1969.

8. M.D. Haust, R.H. More, H.Z. Movat: The Role of the Smooth Muscle Cells in the Fibrogenesis of Arteriosclerosis. The American Journal of Pathology 37:377, 1960.

9. R. Ross, J. Glomset: Atherosclerosis and the Arterial Smooth Muscle Cells. Science 180:1332-9, 1973.

10. J.F. Mustard: Recent Advances in Molecular Pathology. A Review of Platelet Aggregation, Vascular Injury in Atherosclerosis. Experimental Molecular Pathology 7:366-77, 1967.

11. R.E. Tracy, E.B. Merchant, V. Kao: On the Antigenic Identification of Human Serum Beta and Alpha 2 Lipoprotein and Their Identification in the Aortic Intima. Circulation Research 9:472, 1961.

12. Bruce A. Kotke, M.P. Ravi Suffiah: Pathogenesis of Atherosclerosis. Mayo Clinic Proc. 53:35-48, 1978.

13. Robert W. Wissler, D. Vesselinovitch: Studies of Regression of Advanced Atherosclerosis in Experimental Animals and Man. Annals of the New York Academy of Science, Volume 275, pp. 363-78, 1976.

14. E.N. Terry, L.R. Rowen, R.H. Clauss, M.C. Katz, Walter Redisch: Attempts to Delay Progression in Occlusive Atherosclerosis, Annals of the New York Academy of Science. Volume 275, pp. 379-85, 1976.

15. M.L. Armstrong, E.D. Warner, W.E. Connor: Regression of Coronary Atheromatosis in Rhesus Monkeys. Circulation Research 27:59-67, 1970.

16. Jack Whisnant: Epidemiology of Strokes: Emphasis on Transient Cerebral Ischemic Attacks and Hypertension. Stroke 5:68-70, 1974.

17. S. Katz, A.B. Ford, A.B. Chinn, W.A. Newill: Prognosis After Strokes. Medicine 45:236, 1966.

18. J.P. Whisnant, J.P. Fitzgibbon, L.T. Kurland, G.P. Sayre: Natural History of Stroke in Rochester, Minnesota, 1955-1964. Stroke 2:11-21, 1971.

19. H. Eisenberg, J.T. Morrison, P. Sullivan, F.M. Foote: Cerebrovascular Accidents. JAMA 189:883-8, 1964.

20. R.W. Anderson, A. Demirel, R.J. LeBeau: Natural History of Cerebral Thrombosis. Journal of Chronic Diseases 21:221-30, 1968.

21. G.F. Adams, J.D. Merrett: Prognosis and Survival After Strokes. British Medical Journal 1:309, 1961.

22. J.P. Marquardsen: The Natural History of Internal Carotid Acute Cerebrovascular Disease. Acta Neurologica Scandinavia, Supplement 45, pp. 90-188, 1969.

23. J. Marshall, A.C. Kaeser: Survival After Non-hemorrhagic Cerebrovascular Accidents - A Prospective Study. British Medical Journal 2:73-7, 1961.

24. J. Marshall: A Trial of Long-Term Hypotensive Therapy in Cerebrovascular Disease. Lancet Volume I, pp. 10-12, 1964.

25. Veteran's Administration: Cooperative Study, Group on Antihypertensive Agents. Effects of Treatment on Morbidity in Hypertensives. JAMA 202:1028-34, 1967.

26. A.B. Baker, J.A. Resch, R.B. Lowenson: Hypertension and Cerebral Arteriosclerosis. Circulation 39:701-10, 1969.

27. Sylvan Lavy, Eldred Melamed, Esther Cahane, A. Carmon: Hypertension and Diabetes as Risk Factors in Stroke Patients. Stroke 4:751-9, 1973.

28. Veteran's Administration: Cooperative Study, Group on Antihypertensive Agents. Effects of Treatment on Morbidity in Hypertensives. JAMA 202:1028-34, 1967.

29. Veteran's Administration: Effect on Treatment on Morbidity in Hypertension, II Results in Patients with Diastolic Blood Pressure Averaging 90 Through 114 Millimeters of Mercury. JAMA 204:165, 1968.

30. E.D. Freis: Age, Race, Sex and Other Indices of Risk in Hypertension. American Journal of Medicine 55:275-80, 1973.

31. W.B. Kannel, F.W. Blaisdell, R. Gifford, W. Hass, F. McDowell, J.S. Meyer: Risk Factors in Stroke Due to Cerebral Infarction. Stroke 2:423-28, 1971.

32. J.A. Acheson: Factors Affecting the Natural History of Focal Cerebrovascular Disease. Quarterly Journal of Medicine 40:25-46, 1971.

33. William B. Kannel, T.R. Dawber, Paul Sorlie, Phillip Wolf: Comparison of Blood Pressure and Risk of Atherothrombotic Brain Infarction: The Framingham Study. Stroke 7:327-32, 1976.

34. C.M. Fisher: Lacuns: Small Deep Cerebral Infarction. Neurology 15:774, 1965.

35. C.M. Fisher: The Arterial Lesion Underlying Lacuns. Acta Neuropath (Berlin) 12:1, 1969.

36. C.M. Fisher, A.B. Curry: Pure Motor Hemiplegia of Vascular Origin. Archives of Neurology 13:30, 1965.

37. C.M. Fisher: Pure Sensory Stroke Involving Face, Arm, and Leg. Neurology 15:76, 1965.

38. C.M. Fisher, M. Cole: Homolateral Ataxia and Crural Paresis. Journal of Neurology, Neurosurgery, and Psychiatry 28:4, 1965.

39. C.M. Fisher: Lacunar Stroke, The Dysarthria - Clumsy Hand Syndrome. Neurology 17:614, 1967.

40. F.M. Cole, P.O. Yates: Comparative Incidence of Cerebrovascular Lesions in Normotensive and Hypertensive Patients. Neurology 18:255, 1968.

41. B.S. Bansal, C. Prakash, R.K. Arya, S.K. Gulati, S.C. Mettal: Serum Lipid, Platelets, and Fibrinolytic Activity in Cerebrovascular Disease. Stroke 9:137-40, 1978.

42. J. Dyerberg, H.O. Bang, E. Stoffersen, S. Moncada, J.R. Vane: Eicosapentaenoic Acid and Prevention of Thrombosis and Atherosclerosis. Lancet, Volume II, pp. 117-19, 1978.

43. P.J. Palumbo, E.R. Buoner, R.A. Nelson: High Fiber Diet in Hyperlipemia. JAMA 240:223-27, 1978.

44. A.P. Heyman, M.D. Nefzger, E.H. Estes: Serum Cholesterol Levels in Cerebral Infarction. Archives of Neurology 5:264-8, 1961.

45. S. Rossner, K.G. Kgellin, K.L. Mettinger, A. Siden, C.F. Soderstrom: Normal Serum Cholesterol but Low High Density Lipoprotein Cholesterol Concentrations in Young Patients with Ischemic Cerebrovascular Disease. Lancet, Volume I, pp. 577-9, 1978.

46. A.P. Fletcher, Norman Alkjaersig, Andrew Davies, Martin Lewis, John Brooks, William Hardin, William Landau, Marcus Raichle: Blood Coagulation and Plasma Fibrinolytic Enzymes System Pathophysiology in Stroke. Stroke 7:337-48, 1976.

47. Lawrence O. Pilgeram, Anthony N. Chee, Glenn VonDem Bussche: Evidence for Abnormalities in Clotting and Thrombolysis As A Risk Factor for Stroke. Stroke 4: 643-58, 1973.

48. A.T. Masi, M. Dugdale: Cerebrovascular Disease Associated with the Use of Oral Contraceptives. A Review of the English Language Literature. Annals of Internal Medicine 72:111, 1970.

49. Collaborative Group for the Study of Stroke in Young Women: Oral Contraceptive and Increased Risk of Cerebral Ischemia or Thrombosis. New England Journal of Medicine 288:871, 1973.

50. A.B. Carter: Hypotensive Therapy in Stroke Survivors. Lancet, Volume I, pp. 485-9, 1970.

51. William Shahani: Adverse Reaction to Intravascularly Administered Contrast Media. American Journal of Radiology 124:145-52, 1975.

52. D.B. Frens, J.H. Petijan, R. Anderson, H.J. DeBlanc, Jr.: Fibromuscular Dysplasia of the Posterior Cerebral Artery: Report of a Case and a Review of the Literature. Stroke 5:161-6, 1974.

53. J.M. Taveras: Multiple Progressive Intracranial Arterial Occlusion. American Journal of Roentgenology 106:235, 1969.

54. N.T. Matthews, J. Abraham, J. Chandy: Cerebral Angiographic Features in Tuberculous Meningitis. Neurology 20:1015, 1970.

55. K. Higashi, M. Hatano, T. Maza: Disease with Abnormal Intracranial Network Complicated With Intracerebral Hematoma. Journal of Neurology, Neurosurgery and Psychiatry 37:365, 1974.

56. R.T. Johnson, E.P. Richardson: The Neurological Manifestation of Systemic Lupus Erythematosus. Medicine 47:337, 1968.

57. W.G. Wolf, W.C. DeVries: Oxygen Toxicity. Annual Review of Medicine 26:203, 1975.

58. Lawrence McHenry, James W. West, Edward S. Cooper, Herbert I. Goldbert, M.E. Jaffe: Cerebral Autoregulation in Man. Stroke 6:695-706, 1974.

59. J.S. Meyer, Y. Fukuuchi, K. Shimazu, T. Ohuchi, A.D. Ericsson: Abnormal Hemisphere Blood Flow and Metabolism in Cerebrovascular Disease. Stroke 3:157-67, 1972.

60. L.C. McHenry, M.E. Jaffe, I. Kawamura, H.I. Goldbert: Effect of Papaverine on Regional Blood Flow in Focal Vascular Disease of the Brain. New England Journal of Medicine 282:1167-70, 1970.

61. J. Gilroy, M.I. Burnhart, J.S. Meyer: Treatment of Acute Stroke with Dextran Forty. JAMA 210:292-8, 1969.

62. B.M. Patten, J. Mendel, G. Bruun, W. Kurtin, S. Carter: Double Blind Study of the Effects of Dexamethasone in Acute Stroke. Neurology 22:377-83, 1972.

63. R.B. Bauer, H. Tellez: Dexamethasone As Treatment in Cerebrovascular Disease. Stroke 4:547-55, 1973.

64. N.T. Matthew, J.S. Meyer, V.M. Rivera, J.Z. Charney, A. Hartman: Double Blind Evaluation of Glycerol Therapy in Acute Cerebral Infarction. Lancet, Volume II, pp. 13727-9, 1972.

65. W.W. Tourtelotte, J.C. Reinglass, T.A. Newkirk: Cerebral Dehydration Action of Glycerol. Clinical Pharmacology in Therapeutics 13:159-71, 1972.

66. D.G. Beevers, M. Hamilton, M.J. Fairman, J.E. Harpur: Antihypertensive Treatment and the Course of Established Cerebrovascular Disease. Lancet Volume I, p. 1407.

67. E. P. Richardson, Jr., P. R. Dodge, Epilepsy in Cerebrovascular Disease. Epilepsia 3:49-74, 1954.

68. The Canadian Cooperative Study Group: A Randomized Trial of Aspirin and Sulfinpyrazone in the Treatment of Strokes. New England Journal of Medicine 299:53-59, 1978.

CHAPTER III:

STROKE IN EVOLUTION

Stroke in evolution is perhaps the topic that is most speculative and least agreed upon in the classification of ischemic cerebrovascular disease. In many articles concerning cerebral infarctions, it is included as a variation of completed stroke. We feel strongly that it should be separated, and we have organized a separate chapter for its discussion because of its importance. In contrast to completed stroke, the neurologic deficit occurs in some type of progressive fashion. It becomes apparent that there are several ways that this progressive stroke can present. The classical description suggests a step-wise progression in neurologic deficit, which occurs over a period of hours to days. There are also a group of patients who have a slow continuous progression in the magnitude and extent of the deficit over hours to days. There is a third group of patients with progressive strokes who have fluctuations in their severity of neurologic deficit and may also have fluctuations in the extent of the deficit. There may be alternate worsening and improvement over the same time course as mentioned in the other subgroups. Other terms which have been applied to these syndromes are progressive stroke, ingravescent stroke, and thrombosis in evolution. The following case will best illustrate what is meant by a stroke in evolution.

A 65-year-old, hypertensive man awoke with no neurologic deficit. About two hours later, while walking across the room in his home, his right leg buckled and he fell to the floor. He was able to get up and continue walking, but his right leg was definitely weak. Because of important commitments, he continued to his office where he had several meetings. About three hours after the initial event, he noticed that he dropped a pencil while writing and was not able to continue with his writing. At this time, his entire right upper extremity was also noted to be weak; it definitely had been normal until this time. He was concerned and was admitted to the hospital where he was found to have a moderate right hemiparesis. On the morning following admission, while speaking to his secretary on the telephone, he suddenly began using words inappropriately.

This is the history of a patient with a carotid artery stroke in evolution in which no attempt was made to alter the course of the illness. It would not have been at all unusual for each symptom to have improved and worsened several times during the course of his illness.

The following patient is one who presents with thrombosis in evolution in the vertebral artery system.

A 60-year-old man fell to the floor as he entered his office. He had a great deal of difficulty getting up and was helped to a chair. He was taken to a hospital where he was found to have dysarthric speech and weakness in both lower extremities. He also had bilateral extensor plantar responses. When the patient was seen three hours later, he was having difficulty swallowing a glass of water; and his speech was dysarthric with a nasal quality. Five hours after his admission to the hospital, the patient complained of double vision and a right intranuclear ophthalmoplegia was noted. When the patient looked to the right, he could not adduct his left eye completely, and there was nystagmus in the right eye. The problem is that there is <u>no time</u> during the course of the thrombosis in evolution where we can be certain that the neurologic deficit has stabilized. In general, if it has been 24 to 36 hours without progression in the carotid system and 48 in the vertebral basilar system, then there is a strong suggestion that we are dealing with a completed stroke.[1]

The differential diagnosis of stroke in evolution includes some of the same entities which were discussed in the chapter of completed stroke.[2, 7, 9] Because of the progressive nature of this problem, the differentiation is sometimes more difficult. Some factors which point toward this diagnosis are a history of previous cerebrovascular disease and cervical bruits over the carotid and the subclavian arteries. Rapid progression over a brief period of time may also be a hint. A subdural hematoma or a brain tumor may be confused with stroke in evolution if the course of the latter is protracted.

A skull x-ray, computerized tomography scan, and lumbar puncture should be done in all patients in order to make this differentiation as quickly as possible. In stroke in evolution, these studies are most often normal. There can be, however, evidence of an infarction on the computerized tomography scan.

It is hypothesized that the pathogenesis of this problem is the propagation of a thrombus in the carotid or basilar arteries.[1, 3, 4] This has not been proven, but there is suggestive evidence that this is the case. In addition to this, it is thought that the fluctuation during the course of some strokes in evolution is related to emboli breaking off from the thrombus in the large arteries. Because of the large vessel involvement, an isotope flow study might be of help in locating a totally occluded carotid artery. Ophthalmodynamometry or other assessment of retinal artery pressure may also help locate an occluded or highly stenotic internal carotid artery. While angiography would definitely locate the intravascular thrombosis, the use of this study is discouraged early in the course of the illness because of the significant chance of increasing the thrombosis and consequently the patient's neurologic deficit.

When we deal with the posterior circulation, there are a few other diagnoses with which stroke in evolution can be confused. Because most of these are related to brain stem compression, the CT scan and lumbar puncture should most often make this differentiation. The lumbar puncture should not be done until after the scan assures us that there is no mass. If the scan is normal, it still might be necessary to do the lumbar puncture, because on occasion chronic meningitis can mimic an evolving stroke. If no CT scan is available, lumbar puncture must also be done using the precautions discussed in the previous chapter. The reason for this assessment of these patients is that we strongly believe that we can alter the course of thrombosis in evolution and that the morbidity from it can be limited.[1, 3, 5] The earlier that anticoagulation with heparin is instituted, the more likely the therapy is to be helpful. Because anticoagulation can have severe complications, we feel that we should carefully select our patients for this type of therapy. In addition to the usual complications of anticoagulation which include retroperitoneal hemorrhage, our patients have an increased risk of intracerebral hemorrhage. This can occur more easily in the area of recent infarction because of damage to the vascular integrity. If, however, there is a suggestion of progression and no major contraindication to anticoagulation, this should be done with intravenous heparin either continuously or intermittently. The Activated Partial Thromboplastic Time should be kept at 2 to $2\frac{1}{2}$ times the normal control value at $3\frac{1}{2}$ hours after a bolus injection of heparin.

In patients who present with an infarction in the vertebral basilar circulation, which is not easily identified as being in the distribution of a major branch of the basilar artery, i.e., vertebral or posterior-inferior cerebellar artery, we advocate anticoagulation with heparin even if neurologic progression has not occurred. This is so because of the high percentage and dire consequences of progression in these patients. We believe that the mortality and morbidity can be decreased by this type of management. We would recommend oral anticoagulation for at least two to three months after the patient is discharged from the hospital if there is no medical contraindication to it. This should be followed by a prolonged course of aspirin in a dose of 600 mg. b.i.d. With recent information available, it appears that aspirin may decrease the patient's chances of having a cerebral infarction, particularly in men.[8] With this type of medical management, we feel that we may be anticoagulating a few patients with completed strokes in order to treat patients with strokes in evolution as early as possible. If we can decrease the mortality and morbidity as we think that we can, this risk appears to be justified. Before discharge from the hospital, all patients with strokes in evolution of the carotid system should be considered for angiography when the neurologic deficit is stable. Obviously, we are more anxious to study patients who have mild deficits than those who have severe deficits. If the neurologic deficit continues to wax and wane despite heparin therapy, carotid angiography is indicated early in order to delineate a lesion which might be corrected by surgery.

The problem of ischemic cerebrovascular disease is a complicated one, and one that has been known for some time. It has a significant impact on our society, and we are beginning to make progress in treating some forms of it. At the present time our treatment of acute cerebral infarction is somewhat unsatisfactory. We have had better success in altering the course of transient ischemic attacks and strokes in evolution. With the interest that is being shown at several institutions, we hope that we are able to report progress in the management of completed strokes in the not too distant future.

CASE STUDIES

CASE 1:

A 39-year-old, white male was seen in my office in November of 1976. He complained of episodes of numbness involving the right arm, right chest, right face and right leg. These episodes would last from five to ten minutes and they were often relieved by moving his extremities. On one occasion he thought that he might have had numbness in his left arm but he was not sure. These symptoms continued and have been present for approximately one year, averaging about one to two per month. He denied any history of high blood pressure, heart disease or diabetes mellitus.

Systemic neurological review was essentially negative. He has been drinking twelve glasses of beer a day for several years.

Detailed neurological examination was within normal limits. There were no neck bruits present. X-ray of the skull was normal. The electroencephalogram was normal.

It was felt that the patient was suffering from transient ischemic attacks involving the left internal carotid artery system and he was placed on aspirin 650 mg. twice a day. In view of his age, we felt that he had to be watched closely to be certain that the diagnosis was correct.

Despite the aspirin therapy, the episodes of recurrent numbness persisted. From January 1977 to August 1977, he had a total of five recurrent episodes of numbness involving the right lower forearm, right hand and the right chest. We felt that the repetitive episodes of numbness could represent focal jacksonian seizures and he was placed on a therapeutic trial of Dilantin 400 mg. daily. A CT scan was done at this time and without intravenous Conray and it was completely normal.

In October 1977, despite the Dilantin therapy, he had a clonic focal seizure involving the right arm which lasted for about five minutes. He was seen several days later in the office and the neurological examination revealed a fixed deficit consisting of right central facial paresis, mild weakness in the right arm, and a very mild anomic aphasia.

Electroencephalogram at that time showed some theta slowing in the left cerebral hemisphere.

The focal convulsive seizure followed by a fixed neurological deficit suggested the possibility of a left frontal mass lesion and he was subsequently admitted to the hospital in December 1977. The left carotid arteriogram was done at that time and revealed total occlusion of the left internal carotid artery at the carotid siphon intracranially. There was minimal colateral circulation through the external carotid system and through the anterior choroidal artery.

Repeat Computerized Tomography Scan done at that time showed a left frontal infarct. Spinal fluid examination was normal. The electrocardiogram was normal. The CBC and urinalysis and SMA-12 were all within normal limits.

In the hospital, the patient's aphasia became more severe

and he had difficulty completing even the simplest sentences. In view of the progressive neurological deficit in his speech problem, we elected to proceed with an external carotid middle cerebral artery anastomosis. This was done in an attempt to improve the circulation to the left middle cerebral artery system and hopefully to prevent progressive aphasia. The right carotid arteriogram was done prior to the surgery and this study was completely within normal limits. There was good collateral filling from the right carotid circulation to the left through the circle of Willis.

The bypass surgery was carried out with anastomosis of the superficial temporal artery to a branch of the middle cerebral artery on the left side. Both arteries were small but the procedure was completed in a satisfactory manner.

He tolerated the procedure well, but his aphasia and neurological deficit did not change.

He was seen for re-evaluation in my office in March 1978. He had been on aspirin therapy 650 mg. twice a day since discharge from the hospital. He was readmitted to the hospital. At the time of this admission, there was a slight increase in his neurological deficit characterized by increased weakness and spasticity in the right arm. The right central facial paresis was the same and the aphasic disorder was unchanged. It was apparent at that time that the vascular bypass surgery had not been of significant help. A repeat left carotid arteriogram was carried out; this revealed complete thrombosis in the anastomosis between the middle cerebral artery branch and the superficial temporal artery.

This case represents a patient presenting with multiple transient ischemic attacks in the left internal carotid artery system which were not stopped by oral aspirin. Subsequently, he developed a focal clonic seizure involving the right arm which suggested the presence of a left cerebral mass lesion. His neurological deficit progressed slowly and at no time did we have any evidence of a step-like progression. At the time of admission to the hospital for arteriography, it was felt that he had a left frontal mass lesion. Subsequent studies confirmed the diagnosis of a complete occlusion of the internal carotid artery at the carotid siphon. There is no doubt that the slow progression of the neurological deficit represented a thrombosis in evolution involving the left internal carotid artery system. Unfortunately, the middle cerebral artery-external carotid artery bypass surgery was unsuccessful in improving the patient's neurological symptoms. This latter surgery is being done under experimental conditions over wide areas in the United States, to determine if it will be effective in the future.

::

CASE 2:

A 68-year-old, white male was admitted to the hospital at 11 a. m. On arising that morning, he was aware of weakness in the right arm. He had difficulty coordinating movements of the right arm and felt that it was significantly weaker than the left. Past history revealed that he had a similar episode two months ago which lasted about fifteen minutes and disappeared spontaneously. He denied a history of high blood pressure, heart disease or diabetes. He was right handed.

On examination he was alert and oriented with no evidence of aphasia. His right arm drifted downward from the prime outstretched position. There was mild diffuse weakness in all muscles of the right arm compared to the left. There was no weakness in the lower extremities. Rapid repeated movements were slower in the right arm than in the left arm. He hopped normally with both legs. There was a mild right central facial paresis. The remainder of the cranial nerves were intact and there were no field cuts noted. Sensory examination to all modalities was negative. There were no cerebellar abnormalities noted. There were no neck bruits present. The blood pressure was 130/85 in the right arm and 130/80 in the left arm. There was normal sinus rhythm with a rate of 90 per minute. No heart murmurs were heard. The peripheral pulses were normal.

At the time of admission, we felt that the original attack lasted fifteen minutes and represented a transient ischemic attack of the left carotid system. The present attack could represent a transient ischemic attack or could represent a completed stroke, but we felt that the patient should be followed carefully. On the day of admission, the skull x-ray was normal. Chest x-ray was normal. Electrocardiography was normal. SMA-12 was also normal. Lumbar puncture was done and was completely within normal limits, i. e.; the pressure, cell count, protein and serology. Oculoplethysmography was carried out and revealed a thirty percent decrease in the arterial pressure in the left eye as compared to the right eye. We felt that this suggested significant stenosis in his left internal carotid artery despite the fact that no bruits were present. The following day his right arm became weaker and he was watched closely during the next 24 hours. A CT scan that was done at that time showed evidence of a small area of decreased density in the white matter of the left frontal lobe which did not enhance, and we thought it represented a small infarct. The patient had been placed on aspirin at 650 mg. twice a day at the time of his admission. We were concerned that the weakness in the right arm had become progressively worse the following day and he was immediately placed on heparin, after it was determined that his coagulation studies were normal. Heparin was given q4h as a bolus, keeping the APTT at 2 to $2\frac{1}{2}$ times the normal control value. During the next 24 hours, the weakness in his right arm varied from hour to hour. Sometimes his arm was weaker and sometimes it was stronger, but at no time did it improve beyond the original weakness noted at the time of admission. He never developed any involvement in his right lower extremity or his speech. Over the next two days, the variation in weakness in the right arm persisted and we felt that we were unable to stabilize the condition with intravenous heparin. At this time our diagnosis was thrombosis in evolution involving the left internal carotid artery system; we felt that this was confirmed by the decrease in retinal artery pressure on OPG study. Subsequently, a carotid arteriogram was carried out through the femoral approach via catheter. This revealed an ulcer in the internal carotid artery on the left with a large thrombus extending from the ulcer up the internal carotid artery for about two inches. The thrombus was wide and appeared to significantly obstruct the flow of blood through that vessel. It was our feeling that the patient was throwing off emboli from the distal end of this clot which was causing the episodic changes in weakness in his right arm. The patient was immediately taken to the operating room, and the clot and ulcer were removed from the internal carotid artery system via an internal bypass operation. Over the next 48 hours, his condition stabilized and the weakness in the right arm returned to the level that was present on the day of admission. The right carotid artery was studied at the time of the original arteriogram and was within normal limits.

The patient was kept in the hospital for four more days, and his neurological condition appeared to be stable. He was discharged on 650 mg. of aspirin twice a day.

This represented a case with an initial transient ischemic attack, followed by what looked like a completed stroke, followed by what was clearly a thrombosis in evolution involving the left internal carotid artery system. The pathology present at the time of surgery clearly indicates the reasons for the repetitive symptomatology described above.

CASE 3:

A 65-year-old white male, chronic alcoholic, was admitted to the hospital about 12 noon. The previous day he became aware of a sudden onset of an ataxic gait which persisted until he came to the emergency room of the hospital and was subsequently admitted. The patient had no alcohol on his breath at the time of admission. He states that he had been drinking a pint of liquor a day for about ten years. When seen in the emergency room he had a mildly dysarthric speech. Neurological examination revealed vertical nystagmus on upward gaze only. The optic fundi were normal. Cranial nerves were otherwise intact. There was a short soft bruit above the middle of the left clavicle unassociated with a thrill. There were no other neck bruits present. The blood pressure was 230/120 in the left arm and 220/120 in the right arm. Electrocardiogram showed evidence of a left ventricular hypertrophy and strain with normal sinus rhythm. There were no murmurs present.

There was mild appendicular ataxia in the left arm and left leg. There were bilateral Babinski signs. There were no sensory changes present. The patient had been on Aldomet, 250 mg. twice a day and he was continued on this medication. SMA-12 was done and was completely within normal limits. Coagulation studies including prothrombin time, bleeding time, and APTT were normal. Chest x-ray was normal. General physical exam was normal; the liver was not enlarged.

The patient was admitted to the hospital and was seen on rounds about two hours later. At this time, he complained of double vision and he had evidence of internuclear ophthalmoplegia on the left lateral gaze. The left eye deviated to the left with unilateral nystagmus but there was no adduction of the right eye on left lateral gaze. Right lateral gaze was completely normal. At this time, he complained spontaneously of perioral numbness.

A spinal tap was done revealing normal pressure, cell count, protein and serology. We felt the patient was suffering from a stroke involving the vertebral basilar artery system. Since this did not follow the distribution of the posterior inferior cerebellar, anterior-inferior cerebellar artery, superior cerebellar artery or a paramedian branch, we felt that anticoagulation therapy was indicated to prevent any progression in his neurological deficit. Despite the fact that the patient was significantly hypertensive, intravenous heparin was started. The family was given informed consent that the intravenous heparin could lead to hemorrhagic infarct, but we felt that the risk was justified. The neurological deficit stablized, and 40 hours later the patient's Aldomet was increased to 250 mg. four times a day. Prior to the institution of the increased dose of Aldomet, the patient's blood pressure had dropped to 160/95 in both arms. At the time of admission, he was given intravenous Thiamine which was not of any benefit in improving his neurological symptoms.

At the time of discharge three weeks later, the patient continued to have a wide-based gait but was able to balance himself quite well. There were no remaining appendicular cerebellar signs. The Babinski signs, internuclear ophthalmoplegia and nystagmus had disappeared. He was discharged on Coumadin which was to be continued for about one month and then he would be started on aspirin at the dose of 650 mg. twice a day.

This is an example of a patient who had unequivocal evidence of occlusive disease in his vertebral basilar system. Intravenous heparin was started despite the fact that we could not demonstrate definite evidence of thrombosis in evolution.

REFERENCES

1. C.H. Millikan: Reassessment of Anticoagulant Therapy in Various Types of Occlusive Cerebrovascular Disease. Stroke 2:201-208, 1971.

2. E. Clarke and P. Harris: Thrombosis of the Internal Carotid Artery Simulating an Intracranial Space-Occupying Lesion. Lancet, Volume I, pp. 1085-89, 1958.

3. A.B. Carter: Anticoagulant Therapy in Progressing Stroke. British Medical Journal 2:72-73, 1961.

4. R.N. Baker, J.A. Baroward, H.C. Fang, C.M. Fisher, S.N. Groch, A. Heyman, H.R. Karp, E. McDevitt, P. Scheinberg, W. Schwartz, J.F. Toole: Anticoagulant Therapy in Cerebral Infarction. Neurology 12:823-35, 1962.

5. C.M. Fisher: The Use of Anticoagulants in Cerebral Thrombosis. Neurology 8:311-32, 1958.

6. W. McKissock, A. Richardson, L. Walsh: Results of the Surgical Treatment in 244 Consecutive Cases. Lancet, Volume II, pp. 683-86, 1959.

7. W.G. Hardy, D.W. Lindner, L.M. Thomas, E.S. Gurdjian: Anticipated Clinical Course in Carotid Artery Occlusion. AMA, Archives of Neurology 6:138-45, 1962.

8. The Canadian Cooperative Study Group: A Randomized Trial of Aspirin and Sulfinpyrazone in Threatened Strokes. New England Journal of Medicine 299:53-59, 1978.

9. A.B. Carter: Ingravescent Cerebral Infarction. Quarterly Journal of Medicine 29:611-25, 1960.

CHAPTER IV:

CEREBRAL EMBOLI OF CARDIAC ORIGIN

INTRODUCTION

This chapter will deal exclusively with cerebral emboli of cardiac origin. The definitive diagnosis is important because the ultimate therapy will often be different than that used for transient ischemic attacks, completed strokes, and thrombosis in evolution.

The primary approach to the diagnosis is to establish the heart as the source of the cerebral ischemic episode. Certain types of cardiac diseases are frequently associated with cerebral emboli.[1]

NONINFECTED EMBOLI

Rheumatic heart disease with mitral or aortic valvular disease with or without atrial fibrillation may cause cerebral emboli. The patient may give a history of previous rheumatic carditis or may, on examination, have the appropriate murmurs associated with damaged valves secondary to rheumatic fever. Any patient under the age of fifty, with a sudden onset of focal central nervous system symptoms, should be closely evaluated for the possibility of rheumatic heart disease as the source of the emboli. The emboli can arise from the left atrium secondary to mitral valve disease with or without atrial fibrillation, or can arise from platelet-fibrin emboli that adhere to damaged mitral or aortic valves. These platelet-fibrin emboli subsequently break off and shower the systemic circulation. The emboli will subsequently lodge in the brain, other organs of the body, or peripheral vessels in the extremities.[2, 3]

There is also an increased incidence of cerebral emboli with conversion of atrial fibrillation to a normal sinus rhythm. These patients should be anticoagulated for a period of time before the conversion is attempted.[4, 5]

Once it is documented that the rheumatic valvular disease

is the cause of the cerebral emboli, long-term Coumadin therapy is indicated to prevent recurrent episodes. This medication has been effective. The prothrombin time should be kept between 2 and $2\frac{1}{2}$ times the normal control value.

Prosthetic aortic and mitral valves are a common source of cerebral emboli.[6] Platelet-fibrin clots form on the prosthesis and subsequently embolize to the systemic circulation.[7] Cardiac surgeons continue to improve the types of artificial valves used in an attempt to decrease the incidence of embolism.[8] At the present time, pig valves appear to have the least embolic complications. Cardiac surgeons recommend Coumadin or Coumadin with Persantine at the dose of 400 mg. a day to decrease the platelet adhesiveness so that platelet-fibrin clots will not form on the heart valves.[9,10]

Myocardial infarcts, particularly the large infarcts, involving the left ventricle are a source of cerebral emboli. The endocardium is damaged and, subsequently, a mural thrombus forms which will later be the source of the cerebral emboli. The damaged part of the left ventricle is adynamic, and the roughened endocardium serves as a nidus for the clot. This type of infarct probably accounts for most of the emboli that occur within days or weeks of the initial myocardial infarction. Later, with scarring of the ventricle, a ventricular aneurysm or pseudo-aneurysm can form. This will serve as a nidus for the mural thrombosis on the endocardial lining. With congestive heart failure and slowing of the cardiac circulation, there is increased chance of the mural thrombus forming on a damaged endocardium. These are the cases in which an embolism can occur months or years after a myocardial infarct.[11,12] If a cardiac evaluation suggests a strong possibility of endocardial damage and of mural thrombosis, anticoagulation therapy is indicated in an attempt to prevent a clot from forming.

Arteriosclerotic heart disease with chronic atrial fibrillation or intermittent atrial fibrillation can be a source of cerebral emboli.[13] This problem often occurs in elderly patients and in general, it is impossible to differentiate whether the cerebral ischemic episode was related to cardiac embolus, platelet-fibrin clots from carotid lesions or a primary thrombosis of the vessels of the brain. The incidence of strokes in these patients with chronic or intermittent atrial fibrillations is about nine times a control age population. It seems clear that we have underestimated cardiac emboli as a cause of these strokes. Unless the patient has clear evidence of carotid atherosclerosis, these patients should be anticoagulated with Coumadin on a long-term basis.

Surgery on the heart involving the aortic and mitral valves together with open heart surgery and cardiopulmonary bypasses are a frequent source of cerebral emboli. The latter may be due to air, fat, silicone, calcium, or platelet-fibrin clots.[8]

Cerebral emboli also can occur with congenital heart disease, particularly those with right-to-left shunts.[14] They occasionally occur in patients with cyanotic heart disease. Paradoxical emboli sometimes occur in patients with atrial septal defects. Previous pulmonary emboli occur from peripheral venous thrombosis. These emboli lodge in the lungs producing increased right heart pressure. When the right heart pressure exceeds the left heart pressure, emboli are forced from the right atrium into the left atrium and then into the systemic circulation. Paradoxical emboli are also reported with ventricular septal defects.

Atrial myxoma is an uncommon cause of cerebral emboli.[15] The diagnosis is to be considered in any young patient with symptoms compatible with a cerebral or peripheral emboli. The most common location for the tumor is in the left atrium. Pieces of the tumor can break off and embolize in the systemic circulation. Sometimes a diagnosis is made when the embolus is removed surgically from a peripheral artery. The myxoma can obstruct the flow of blood in the left atrium producing symptoms related to acute increase in pulmonary pressure. The myxoma can also produce chest pains, heart murmurs, and cardiac arrhythmias. A high index of suspicion will lead to appropriate diagnostic tests, such as echocardiogram and/or cardiac angiography. Removal of the tumor by surgery is the treatment of choice.

Recently there have been some papers discussing prolapse of the mitral valve in young patients, as a source of cerebral emboli.[16] These patients can have recurrent chest pains and cardiac arrhythmias. Sometimes auscultation reveals a mid-systolic click. Echocardiogram will demonstrate the prolapsed mitral valve. The emboli arise from platelet-fibrin clots that adhere to the prolapsed valve. At the present time, the treatment of choice is the use of platelet antagonists. This etiology will require further evaluation because many patients have prolapsed mitral valves without associated adverse symptoms.[17]

Patients with cardiac myopathies that are often related to chronic alcoholism, can embolize because of irregularities in the endocardium associated with congestive heart failure.

Also, patients with congestive heart failure, enlarged left ventricle and atrium can embolize with supraventricular and ventricular arrhythmias.

Nonbacterial thrombotic endocarditis (marantic endocarditis) is associated with carcinoma. The vegetations on the heart valves are of platelet-fibrin origin. This entity represents a partial form of disseminated intravascular coagulopathy. It is most often seen with mucin-secreting carcinomas. The combination of carcinoma, peripheral thrombophlebitis, and cerebral embolism should lead to the correct diagnosis and avoid the erroneous diagnosis of metastatic carcinoma to the brain.[1]

INFECTED EMBOLI

Patients with bacterial endocarditis present a different clinical problem because the emboli contain viable bacteria. The differentiation of acute from subacute bacterial endocarditis is related to the virulence of the bacteria. The infection can occur on damaged heart valves, prosthetic heart valves, or on congenital heart defects.[18,19,20]

Patients can present with many different clinical patterns:

a) Meningismus

b) Toxic psychosis (elderly)

c) Encephalitis or cerebritis

d) Subarachnoid hemorrhage (mycotic aneurysm)

e) Brain abscess

f) Sudden onset of focal central nervous system signs

The infected emboli lodge in the cerebral arteries often in a distal location close to the cortex. This can produce a pleocytosis in the spinal fluid with associated headache, photophobia and nuchal rigidity. These patients present with a suspected diagnosis of meningitis. When the emboli are multiple, the patients can become aphasic, confused, disoriented and are febrile. These symptoms together with the spinal fluid changes can lead to an erroneous diagnosis of viral encephalitis. In elderly people, fever from any source can often produce a toxic psychosis that is associated with visual hallucinations, confusion and delirium. These patients should always be carefully evaluated for associated cardiac disease.

When the infected emboli lodge in the larger arteries, the patient develops a sudden onset of focal neurological deficits. These deficits are often less complete than those associated with total occlusions of the internal carotid or middle cerebral artery systems. Patients can develop a monoparesis instead of hemiparesis, quadrantic defect on the visual fields instead of hemianopic defect, and partial sensory changes in any extremity. The presence of cortical infarcts associated with emboli often lead to convulsive seizures, both the focal and generalized type. After the infected emboli is lodged in the artery or vaso vasorum, it can weaken the arterial wall and lead to a mycotic aneurysm. Subsequent rupture of the aneurysm will lead to a subarachnoid hemorrhage.

With acute endocarditis, because of the virulent organisms involved, patients can develop multiple small brain abscesses.

The spinal fluid pressure can be normal and slightly elevated. The pleocytosis can vary from no cells to hundreds of cells depending upon the organism involved. The cells can be mostly polys in acute bacterial endocarditis or mostly lymphocytes in subacute bacterial endocarditis. The protein is elevated but usually less than 100 mg.%. The cerebral spinal fluid sugar is normal in subacute bacterial endocarditis but can be decreased in acute bacterial endocarditis. With subarachnoid hemorrhages, the spinal fluid is grossly bloody and under increased pressure.

The diagnosis of bacterial endocarditis will depend upon a cardiac evaluation suggesting chronic valvular disease, prosthetic valves, or congenital heart disease. A heart murmur that was not previously present should suggest acute bacterial endocarditis. The valvular defects can be confirmed by auscultation and by echocardiogram. The ultimate diagnosis comes from a positive culture of the offending organism. It should be noted in passing that endocarditis rarely occurs with organisms other than bacteria.

Patients are to be treated with appropriate antibiotics necessary to eradicate the infection in the blood and on the heart valves. The earlier therapy is started, the better the results. With early diagnosis and appropriate treatment, the patients are less likely to develop mycotic aneurysms or cerebral abscesses. In certain instances the infection cannot be eradicated on prosthetic valves; under these circumstances, the valves must be removed and replaced by new valves. Anticoagulation therapy with Coumadin is not indicated with endocarditis and infected emboli because of possible subarachnoid hemorrhage. The primary physician or internist can often make the appropriate diagnosis when a patient presents with cerebral embolism, peripheral embolism, and heart disease associated with a febrile course.

THE NEUROLOGICAL APPROACH TO CEREBRAL EMBOLISM

A neurologist approaches the diagnosis of cerebral emboli in certain different ways. He is aware that finding the cardiac source is of prime importance. He is also aware that the presence of peripheral embolic phenomena to the spleen, kidney, liver, and peripheral arteries helps make the diagnosis easier. However, the neurologist can often suspect emboli from evaluation of the brain alone. In the brain he searches for multiple lesions. Sometimes this can be done clinically by demonstrating focal ischemic changes in both hemispheres, or by the demonstration of lesions both above and below the tentorium.

Radioactive brain scans sometime demonstrate the presence of multiple lesions, and when associated with cardiac disease, the diagnosis would appear certain.

Computerized axial tomography is more effective than radioactive brain scans in demonstrating multiple lesions of the brain, both above and below the tentorium.[21] These lesions are often white or ischemic infarcts. However, the presence of multiple hemorrhagic infarctions is highly suggestive of a diagnosis of cerebral emboli.[22] With computerized tomography scanning, it is better to wait from 4 to 7 days after the stroke before carrying out the procedure. This delay will allow for better visualization of the cerebral infarcts. Increased density around the infarcts, due to capillary bleeding, in the unenhanced scan near or in the cortex is suggestive of a hemorrhagic infarct. As alluded to previously, hemorrhagic infarcts are most commonly associated with cerebral emboli. After dye enhancement, some of the infarcts will "light up", therefore making it easier to see multiple lesions.

Hemorrhagic infarcts often produce microscopic or gross blood in the cerebral spinal fluid. To best demonstrate the red blood cells in the spinal fluid, one should wait from 24 to 48 hours after the ictus before the lumbar puncture is performed. This will allow time for the red blood cells to migrate from the brain to the lumbar subarachnoid space.

Seizures are most common with cerebral emboli and less common with nonembolic strokes; this is because the small emboli particles often lodge in the cortical arteries. The seizures can be focal or grand mal in type and can precede or come shortly after the focal neurological deficit.

The emboli lodge in the carotid system more often than the vertebral basilar system. The left carotid system is more often embolized than the right. The neurological profile of cerebral emboli of cardiac origin consists of:

1) the sudden onset of focal brain deficit reaching maximum intensity in minutes

2) focal or generalized seizures

3) microscopic or gross red blood cells in the spinal fluid (fifty red blood cells or more)

4) multiple lesions noted clinically or by radioactive isotope scanning or by computerized axial tomography

5) the presence of hemorrhagic infarct on computerized tomography scanning

6) most frequent involvement in the left carotid artery system

The convulsive seizure should be treated with intravenous Phenobarbital, with the dose depending on the age of the patient and the frequency of the seizures. If it is necessary for the patient to be given Dilantin rapidly, the patient should be given 1000 mm. intravenously at the rate of 50 mg. per minute. This drug has the advantage of not producing drowsiness. It should be used if reasonable doses of Phenobarbital do not stop the seizures. If the patient is 65 or older, the dose of Phenobarbital should be 100 mg. given intravenously. If this does not stop the seizures, then the patient can be given intravenous Dilantin as described above. If the patient is in a young age group from 30 to 50, the dose of Phenobarbital should be 250 mg. intravenously; and if this does not stop the seizures, the dosage should be repeated. If the seizures do not stop, then intravenous Dilantin is indicated. Dilantin is to be used with caution in patients with cardiac arrythmias. When Phenobarbital is used one must be prepared to intubate if respiratory arrest occurs.

Valium, intravenously, can stop a seizure but is not a good anticonvulsant and must be supplemented with phenobarbital or Dilantin.

As discussed previously, anticoagulation therapy is the treatment of choice to prevent repetitive emboli in most cases. This therapy should be held in abeyance until the computerized tomography scan and the lumbar puncture are done to rule out the presence of hemorrhagic infarcts. If these tests show the presence of hemorrhagic infarcts or blood in the spinal fluid, anticoagulation therapy should not be started for one week, and then it should be started with Coumadin and not heparin.[23] The exception is if the emboli are multiple and life-threatening. If there is no evidence of hemorrhage infarct or red blood cells in the spinal fluid, IV Heparin can be started acutely or if the physician prefers Coumadin.

The primary physician is in an excellent position to anticipate which cardiac problems can lead to emboli. When the risk factor is high, appropriate medical or surgical therapy is indicated to prevent cerebral emboli and associated catastrophic central nervous system deficits.

CASE STUDIES

CASE 1:

A 51-year-old white male was at home having dinner with his family about 6:30 p. m.; they suddenly became aware that he was having difficulty with his speech. He had trouble understanding what was being said to him, and his responses to the family were garbled and inappropriate. The patient was right-handed, and the family was not aware of any weakness of his extremities. He went to lay down on the couch, and within a half an hour, his speech had improved but he still had difficulty coming up with appropriate words in his sentence structure. Despite the objections of the patient, the family took him to the emergency room where he was seen at approximately 8:00 p. m.

At this time, he was alert and oriented. Careful testing of his speech did not reveal any evidence of aphasia. The neurological examination was completely negative. There were no neck bruits present. The blood pressure was 130/85 in both arms.

At this time, it was felt he had a transient ischemic attack of his left internal carotid artery system producing the aphasic reaction described in the history. Electrocardiogram taken in the emergency room showed an old large anterolateral ventricular infarct, with occasional unifocal premature ventricular contractions; the rate was 90 per minute. On close questioning, the patient denied ever having a history of heart disease, angina pectoris, or previous myocardial infarction. He was never aware of palpitations, congestive failure, or any other type of arrhythmia. In view of the ventricular premature beats, he was admitted to the coronary care unit so that his cardiac status would be monitored. Careful questioning in the unit failed to reveal any previous episodes to suggest transient ischemic attacks of the vertebral basilar or the carotid artery system. The patient was placed on aspirin at the dose of 650 mg. twice a day. No specific therapy was given for the unifocal premature ventricular contractions. CBC and urinalysis were negative. SMA-12 consisting of blood sugar, BUN, creatinine, uric acid, cholesterol, CO_2, chlorides, sodium, potassium, calcium, alkaline phosphatase, and SGOT were all within normal limits. CPK was normal. Chest x-ray was normal and did not reveal any significant cardiac enlargement. The following day the patient was seen in consultation by the cardiologist who felt that the patient had a significant myocardial infarct, and suggested that we carry out cardiac fluoroscopy and echocardiogram. The echocardiogram revealed decrease in the size of the ventricular wall in the area of the infarct. Cardiac fluoroscopy revealed a large area involving the left lateral ventricle which was adynamic during ventricular contraction. The cardiologist felt that the adynamic area in the heart was serving as a nidus for a mural thrombus, which subsequently embolized into his left carotid circulation. Forty-eight hours after admission, a computerized tomography scan was done without intravenous Conray and was completely within normal limits. A spinal fluid examination was normal and did not reveal any microscopic red blood cells. The patient's coagulation studies were also within normal limits. Oculoplethysmography studies failed to reveal any difference in the retinal artery pressures in either eye.

At the request of the cardiologist, the patient was started on intravenous heparin. This medication was continued for a week, and the heparin was subsequently switched to Coumadin therapy. The premature ventricular contractions ceased after he was in the hospital for about one week. Repeat CPK studies were all within normal limits. The plan, after discharge from the hospital was to keep him on the Coumadin therapy for several months; then re-admit him to the hospital for coronary angiography, to determine whether any coronary bypass surgery would be indicated in the future.

This case is an example of cerebral embolism of cardiac origin, in which the symptomatology falls into the classification of a transient ischemic attack, since the aphasia lasted less than twenty-four hours. The case emphasizes the necessity for evaluating the heart as a source for symptoms suggesting either transient ischemic attacks or completed strokes.

::

CASE 2:

A 72-year-old black male was brought to the emergency room. Thirty minutes before, he had collapsed on the street and was brought via a police ambulance. When he was seen in the emergency room, at the time of admission, he was globally aphasic. His eyes were deviated to the left. There was a flaccid paralysis of the right arm and right leg, which was complete. There was a right central facial paresis and a right Babinski sign. The neck was supple, and the optic discs were flat. There were no neck bruits. The patient had evidence of auricular fibrillation with a ventricular rate of 85 per minute. No heart murmurs were heard. The blood pressure varied from 140/90 to 120/80 in both arms. Skull x-ray and chest x-ray were normal. SMA-12 was normal. A complete blood count and urinalysis were normal. The patient was afebrile at the time of admission. Electrocardiogram showed evidence of auricular fibrillation with no evidence of myocardial damage. His private physician was contacted by phone, and he confirmed the fact that, for many years, the patient had auricular fibrillation. We felt the patient had a completed stroke involving the left internal carotid artery system. He was admitted to the intensive care unit. The following morning there was no change in his neurological status except that his neck appeared to be mildly rigid. Computerized tomography scan was done that afternoon and revealed four hemorrhagic infarcts in the left cerebrum, all involving primarily the cortical and subcortical white matter. There was no ventricular shift seen on the CT scan. Lumbar puncture revealed initial pressure of 190 mm. of water. The spinal fluid was grossly bloody in all tubes. There were 12,000 red blood cells, 35 white blood cells, half lymphocytes and half polys and a protein of 65 mg.%.

On the basis of the CT scan, it was our feeling that the patient embolized from his left atrium into the left internal carotid artery system, producing the multiple hemorrhagic infarcts in the left cerebrum. The blood in the spinal fluid, with the clinical findings, suggested an intracerebral hemorrhage. The CT scan was diagnostic for multiple hemorrhagic infarcts.

In view of the blood noted in the spinal fluid, anticoagulation was not started. The patient did not make any significant improvement throughout his hospital course and was transferred to a nursing home for long-term care.

If a computerized tomography scan were not available, the spinal tap would have suggested that the patient had an intracerebral hemorrhage, producing the left cerebral damage. This would have required a carotid arteriogram to rule out a surgically-treated intracerebral bleed.

This case represents a patient with chronic auricular fibrillation who, indeed, did embolize to the left cerebral system. There are certain cases where an embolus cannot be differentiated from a completed stroke, unless the criterion for hemorrhagic infarction are fulfilled by CT scan or lumbar puncture.

CASE 3:

A 38-year-old white male was in perfect health until the day of admission to the hospital. He awoke in the morning and talked to his wife, who was on her way to work. One-half hour later his children called his wife at work to tell her that their father was talking in a confused manner and wandering around the house; they could not understand what he was saying. The wife immediately went home and found the husband in his bed, with evidence of fecal incontinence and a bleeding tongue. At that time, she was aware that he was having a great deal of difficulty with his speech, and he was definitely confused. He was subsequently taken to a local hospital, by ambulance, where examination in the emergency room revealed him to be confused with an organic mental syndrome. They could not document any aphasia at that time, but there seemed little question that he had been aphasic previously. He was admitted to the hospital. Skull x-ray was completely within normal limits. SMA-12 was within normal limits. CBC and urinalysis were normal. Electrocardiogram was normal and chest x-ray was normal.

Several days later a computerized tomography scan was done which revealed a large area of decreased density in the left frontal region. Bilateral carotid arteriogram studies were done, as well as aortic arch studies. These failed to reveal any significant pathology in the carotid arteries in the neck and no evidence of any definite occlusion of his intracranial vessels.

The patient was subsequently transferred to another hospital for further evaluation. Mental status revealed the patient to be moderately demented. He owned his own business, and he was aware that both his mathematics, his recent memory and his general intellectual abilities were diminished; this was confirmed on mental status. There were no focal neurologic findings noted and he was not aphasic. His blood pressure was 120/80 in both arms. Electrocardiogram was normal. Auscultation of the heart revealed a mid-systolic click over the mitral area. Review of the computerized tomography scan confirmed a large area of decreased density in the left frontal lobe representing an infarct, but also showed a small infarct on the right frontal lobe. Lumbar puncture was completely within normal limits as to pressure, cells, protein and serology. Electroencephalogram showed theta slowing in the left frontal lobe.

Coagulation studies were normal. A work-up for vasculitis was completely negative. In view of the changes on CT scan, we felt that the patient had evidence of bilateral cerebral lesions. In view of the multiple lesions present, we felt that the heart must be the source of the infarcts; this seemed logical in the absence of any pathological lesions in the aortic arch and carotid arteries, extracranially and intracranially. An echocardiogram was done, and it revealed a definite prolapse of his mitral valve. Cardiac consultation confirmed the mid-systolic click and echocardiogram confirmed the diagnosis of a prolapsed mitral valve. It would seem that the prolapse of the mitral valve was a source of platelet-fibrin emboli, which caused the ischemic infarctions in the left frontal lobe, and to a lesser extent, the right frontal lobe. There is no doubt that the fecal incontinence and bleeding tongue reflected a grand mal seizure that occurred after the initial period of confusion.

The patient was placed on Phenobarbital, 60 mg. twice a day to prevent recurrent seizures. In addition, he was placed on aspirin, 650 mg. twice a day in an attempt to prevent further platelet-fibrin emboli from accumulating on his prolapsed mitral valve.

This case appears to represent a bona fide example of mitral prolapse with accumulation of platelet-fibrin clots on the valve and subsequent embolization to the brain.

REFERENCES

1. J. Willis Hurst: The Heart, 3rd Edition, McGraw-Hill Book Company, New York, N. Y., 1974.

2. M. Swash and D.J. Earl: Transient Visual Obscurations in Chronic Rheumatic Heart Disease. Lancet, Volume 1, p. 323, 1970.

3. H.S. Weily, P.P. Steele, et al.: Platelet Studies in Patients with Rheumatic Heart Valves. New England Journal of Medicine 290:539, 1974.

4. B. Loun: Electrical Reversion of Cardiac Arrhythmias. British Heart Journal 29:469, 1967.

5. C.J. Bjerhelund and O. Morning: The Efficacy of Anticoagulants in Preventing Pulmonary Embolism Related to Electrical Conversion of Atrial Fibrillation. American Journal of Cardiology 23:208, 1969.

6. M. Akbarian, W.G. Austen, et al.: Thromboembolic Complications of Prosthetic Cardiac Valves. Circulation 37:826, 1968.

7. L.A. Harker and S.J. Slichter: Studies of Platelet and Fibrinogen Kinetics in Patients with Prosthetic Heart Valves. New England Journal of Medicine 283:1302, 1970.

8. A. Starr, R.H. Herr, et al.: Mitral Replacement: Review of Six Years Experience. Journal of Thoracic-Cardiovascular Surgery 54:333, 1967.

9. J.E. Arrants and P. Hairston: Use of Persantine in Preventing Thrombo-embolism Following Valve Replacement. American Surgery 38:432, 1972.

10. G.E. Duvoisin, et al.: Late Results of Cardiac Valve Replacement. Circulation 37:75, 1968.

11. M.D. Klein, M.V. Herman, et al.: A Hemodynamic Study of Left Ventricular Aneurysm. Circulation 35:614, 1967.

12. W.C. Kane, S.M. Aronson: Cardiac Disorders Predisposing to Embolic Stroke. Stroke 1:164, 1970.

13. W. Blackwood, J. F. Hallpike, et al.: Atheromatous Disease of the Carotid Arterial System and Embolism from the Heart in Cerebral Infarction: A Morbid Anatomical Study. Brain 92:897, 1969.

14. R.S. Fontana and J.E. Edwards: Congenital Cardiac Disease - A Review of 357 Cases Studied Pathologically, W.B. Saunders Co., Philadelphia, 1962.

15. W.F. Greenwood: Profile of Atrial Myxoma. American Journal of Cardiology 21:367, 1968.

16. H.J. Barnett, M.W. Jones, et al.: Cerebral Ischemic Events and Prolapsing Mitral Valve. Archives of Neurology 33:777, 1976.

17. O.R. Brown, F.E. Loster, et al.: Incidence of Mitral Valve Prolapse in the Asymptomatic Normal. Circulation 52:77, 1975.

18. R.B. Shaffer, W.D. Hall: Bacterial Endocarditis Following Open Heart Surgery. American Journal of Cardiology 25:602, 1970.

19. R. Vogler and E. Dorney: Bacterial Endocarditis in Congenital Heart Disease. American Heart Journal 64:198, 1962.

20. J. Geraci, A. Dale, et al.: Bacterial Endocarditis and Endarteritis Following Cardiac Operations. Wisconsin Medical Journal 62:302, 1963.

21. J. Masdue, H. Berhooz, et al.: Evaluation of Recent Cerebral Infarction by Computerized Tomography. Archives of Neurology 34:417, 1977.

22. Paul New: Computed Tomography in the Diagnosis of Hemorrhagic Stroke. Stroke 16:145, 1977.

23. J.P. Whisnant, C.H. Millikan, et al.: Effects of Anticoagulants on Experimental Cerebral Infarction; Clinical Implications. Circulation 20:56, 1959.

INDEX

INDEX